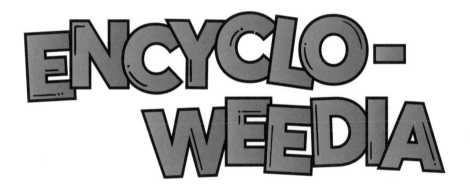

For obvious reasons, and in humble consideration
of our long & affectionate association, the present
volume is dedicated to Spoon.

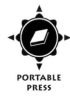

Portable Press
An imprint of Printers Row Publishing Group
9717 Pacific Heights Blvd, San Diego, CA 92121
www.portablepress.com · mail@portablepress.com

Printers Row Publishing Group is a division of
Readerlink Distribution Services, LLC.
Portable Press is a registered trademark of
Readerlink Distribution Services, LLC.

Correspondence regarding the content of
this book should be sent to Portable Press,
Editorial Department, at the above address.
Rights inquiries should be addressed to
HarperCollins*Publishers*, 1 London Bridge Street,
London SE1 9GF, www.harpercollins.co.uk.

Portable Press
Publisher: Peter Norton
Associate Publisher: Ana Parker
Acquisitions Editor: Kathryn C. Dalby

Produced by **HarperCollins***Publishers*
Designer: Abi Read
Author: Jack Kapos
Illustrations: Abi Read

Library of Congress Control Number:
2020946578

ISBN: 978-1-64517-672-5

Printed in Latvia

25 24 23 22 21 1 2 3 4 5

Disclaimer: The material offered in this book is presented for informational and entertainment purposes,
and the publisher has made every effort to ensure the information was correct at press time; however, the
publisher and author make no claims or guarantees whatsoever regarding the accuracy, interpretation,
or utilization of any of the information provided herein. The contents of this book are not an endorsement
of or encouragement to use marijuana, which at this printing is illegal for consumption and use in many
states and remains a Schedule 1 Controlled Substance under U.S. federal law. The contents are not
medical advice or meant to diagnose, treat, cure, or prevent any illness or disease or substitute for the
advice of a health care professional. Portions of this book may describe activities that may be hazardous
or may be illegal in certain states or provinces. The author and publisher do not assume and hereby
disclaim any liability to any party for any loss, damage, or disruption caused by errors, omissions,
or otherwise, which may result from negligence, accident, or any other cause.

JACK KAPOS

ENCYCLO-WEEDIA

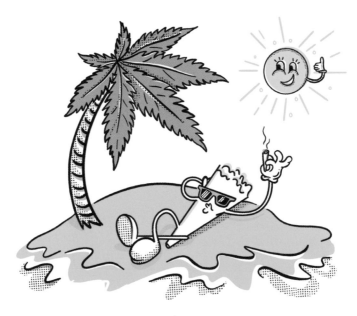

PORTABLE
PRESS

SAN DIEGO, CALIFORNIA

table of CONTENTS

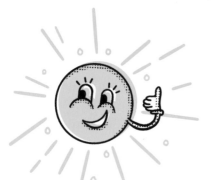

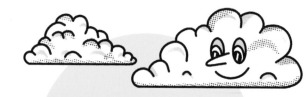

Introduction

"I apprehended music in a new manner under the influence of marijuana, and these apprehensions have remained valid in years of normal consciousness... And I saw anew many of nature's panoramas & landscapes that I'd stared at blindly without even noticing before; thru the use of marijuana, awe & detail were made conscious."

Allen Ginsberg: *Poet, voice of a generation, smoker*

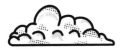

It's easy for our weed use to become a comfortable corner of our lives: that moment of calm at the end of the day when we settle down, skin up, and take a soothing pull on a joint. And there's nothing wrong with that.

But what if it became the key to living life to the fullest, as it did for Allen Ginsberg? What if it were the inspiration behind your next cultural discovery, life-changing vacation, spiritual insight, or intellectual revelation? In these pages, you'll discover a host of life-changing ideas, sights, sounds, activities, and destinations, all with their own reefer recommendations to let you get the most from the moment and make memories to treasure. You'll be taken on a journey along the spectrum of bud—from *sativa* to *indica*—and you'll find a host of ways to employ cannabis and enjoy its amazing psychological and health benefits.

There is a serious side, too. We are now starting to enjoy the benefits of drug law liberalization, in the U.S. and around the world, but there is still so much that needs to be done. For every town that has professional legal dispensaries and understanding law enforcement, there is another where innocent enjoyment of the herb can land you in serious trouble.

Inspiring and informative, here are 420 "smokes" that will improve the quality of your life immeasurably, with entries covering techniques, recipes, music, reading, viewing, travel, history, philosophy, and even a guide to using cannabis for better relationships and sex.

Stop being the boring stoner on the couch. This is your chance to become the amazing stoner *everywhere*.

Mercury Rev
Primal Scream
Bob Marley
The Warlocks
D'Angelo
Herbie Hancock
Beastie Boys
Cypress Hill
The Pharcyde
Missy Elliott
Wu-Tang Clan
The Avalanches
Gorillaz
Wiz Khalifa
Nuyorican Soul
DJ Shadow
Daft Punk
Steve Reich
Massive Attack
Flaming Lips
Portishead
Pink Floyd
Grateful Dead
Snoop Dogg
Galaxie 500
Andrew Weatherall
Spiritualized

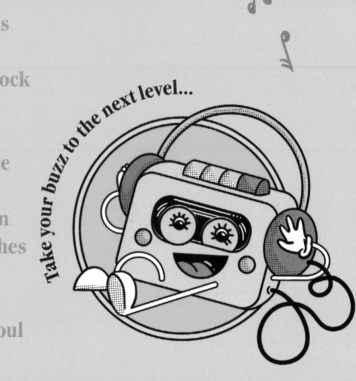

Take your buzz to the next level...

Musical Smokes

The easiest way to add a layer of meaning and complexity to your high is to put on some music.

But what kind is the best for taking your buzz to the next level? Or, looked at the other way, what kind of music is most enhanced by a mellow atmosphere? Does it really matter which way you look at the question anyhow? What's undeniable is that music and marijuana have been intimately intertwined for a hundred years or more—and we all know what kind of song goes best with a toke. The rhythms tend to be pulsing, not frantic; songs don't burst into massive anthemic choruses (power ballads are for beer drinkers), and vocals tend to the downbeat, even melancholy. A groove will unwind over five minutes or more; instruments or vocals will step forward, do their thing, then step back; lyrics, if there are any, can be surreal or repetitious.

The albums celebrated here have been carefully selected to take you on a range of musical journeys. With your mind relaxed and your thoughts free to wander, these performances will unwind, at a leisurely pace, repeating and varying themes, building up before drifting down… So make yourself comfortable, dim the lights, and put yourself into the hands of these expert musicians—many of whom were experienced stoners themselves.

The easiest way to add a layer of meaning and complexity to your high is to put on some music.

A groove will unwind over five minutes or more; instruments or vocals will step forward, do their thing, then step back.

In a silent way

In a Silent Way, Miles Davis

An intense, incredibly serious musician, Miles Davis would have been furious to see this radical masterwork recommended as fantastic music to get stoned to. Too bad: it *is* fantastic music to get stoned to. There are only two tracks, and they abandon altogether the traditional structures of verse and chorus, consisting only of the very loosest grooves, edited together from extensive improvised jams, into which Miles and his band of genius jazzers dip in and out, seemingly at random, yet creating a gravity-free mood of space and time that you'll never forget. This is an intimate journey: a solo smoke, because you won't want to be distracted by the presence of other people.

In C, Terry Riley

Loosely structured and consisting of fifty-three melodic fragments that a flexible number of musicians repeat on a flexible selection of instruments at their own discretion, *In C* will take you on a strange, at times challenging, journey through sound and time. Put any one of its many versions on when you are very comfortably stoned, yet alert, and ready to pick up on tiny details, unexpected rhythms, and new textures.

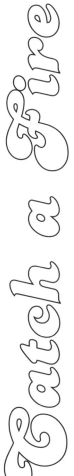

Catch a Fire, **Bob Marley**

Consider even just the cover. This is smoking at its proudest: a sun-drenched Marley looks out at the camera and pulls on a spliff that's some way fatter than his middle finger. The grooves within form one of the finest reggae albums of them all: liquid, flowing rhythms, catchy hooks, and Marley's yearning vocals pulling on your heartstrings all the way through. With no production tricks or dub wizardry, this blend of soul and musicianship perfectly expresses the joyful, melancholy, and spiritual aspects of ganja, the Rastafarians' sacred herb.

UFOrb, **The Orb**

Ambient music is great for smoking. Dub reggae is great for smoking. Comedy records and sound-effects are great for smoking. It was The Orb's genius to mash all of these genres together, creating tracks that could be seventeen minutes long, with hypnotic drum loops, endlessly pulsing reggae basslines, pretty synthesizer lines, and floating over the top… literally *anything*. Animal noises, distant engine sounds, prank calls, the sound of supernovas, all were given a deep, spacey echo and left to play out. This meandering album is the ideal soundtrack to an intimate late-night conversation that promises to solve the problems of the universe. And as you would expect, it is great for smoking.

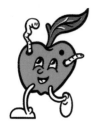

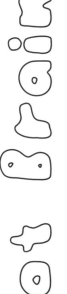

Maggot Brain, Funkadelic

The members of George Clinton's innovative funk-rock powerhouse were heavy weed users, and this early masterpiece is a perfect expression of the many faces of the buzz. The epic guitar instrumental that opens the set juxtaposes a tranquil, looping chord change with a pyrotechnic, echoing solo that will, at the right volume, literally blow your mind. The songs that follow are completely different: catchy vocals, laid-back grooves, and lyrics that—with Funkadelic's trademark anarchic humor—encourage the listener to "Hit it and Quit it" before we all end up "Back in our Minds." This is a *completely* out-there record, and perfect if you happen to have slightly overdone it and need a groove to carry you through to the other side—and back to the party.

Doggystyle, Snoop Dogg

The 1990s was a golden age of laid-back, drawled rap delivered by proud stoners—many of whom were audibly rhyming through that characteristic tight voice box that arrives with a heavy smoking session. Snoop Doggy Dogg, as he was known at the time, defined the genre with 1993's *Doggystyle*: languid lyrical delivery over some of Dr. Dre's catchiest grooves—many of which owed a debt to George Clinton's P-Funk pioneers. Laid-back while still working hard, this is a record that makes you feel like you're dancing even as you remain rooted to the couch. It was the start of a long, relaxed career for Snoop, a man who is rarely not stoned and claims to run on eighty-one blunts a day.

Selected Ambient Works 85–92, Aphex Twin

Much of this album was recorded at home when Aphex Twin (Richard James) was still in his teens, and its muffled, tape-recorded quality betrays its low-budget, self-engineered origins. Don't be betrayed, though, this album was packed with ideas and is universally recognized as a landmark in techno, ambient, and dance music. Synth bass squelches, kick drums pulse, melodies drift in and out, and the tracks drift from soundscape to soundscape, but the album never drags, and it's full of hooks, tunes, textures, and rhythms that remain surprising to this day. Even the track names ("Xtal," "Tha," "Schottkey 7th Path") are like nothing else. Put it on, add your own smoke to the mix, and let the Twin do the rest.

John Coltrane & Johnny Hartman, John Coltrane and Johnny Hartman

Jazz never sounded smokier than on this record of romantic standards, recorded in one session by John Coltrane, one of jazz's great names, and Hartman, a little-known ballad specialist. In only six songs, the pair conjure a mellow feel that's never been bettered: smooth and sentimental, but never saccharine, and full of spontaneity and subtle detail. Put this on for a late-night smoke with your loved one and be seduced alternately by Hartman's heartfelt baritone voice and Coltrane's plaintive tenor sax. Coltrane never recorded another album with a vocalist. He didn't need to: this one is perfection.

Melodies drift in and out
Melodies drift in and out

Exile on Main St, The Rolling Stones

The product of chaotic recording sessions in the basement of Keith Richards' rented chateau, *Exile* is the sound of a band at their loosest, rawest, and most exhilarating. This double album slides from uptempo rock ("Rip this Joint") to laid-back blues groove ("Turd on the Run") and the grittiest soul ("Shine a Light") and still sounds absolutely whole and unified. Buried in the foggy, indistinct mix (which he complains about to this day, fifty years later) are some of Jagger's best lyrics: wry celebrations of the Stones' travels, troubles, and love lives—and some rueful moans about the difficulties presented by Keith Richards' nocturnal, drug-addled, chaotic lifestyle.

YERSELF IS STEAM

Yerself Is Steam, Mercury Rev

While Nirvana were tearing up the charts and REM were the conscience of a generation, Mercury Rev were the alternative rockers who were more interested in the small stuff. Chasing a bee, for instance, or seeing colors—wasting time, in general. It was that attitude that made them less successful than their fuzzy, melodic, indie rock deserved. "I've seen you fritter away/slow as a glacier makes its way down to the Rhine," sings Jonathan Donahue: it's hard to know if he's addressing his stoned and unreliable bandmates, or his stoned and unreliable fanbase.

Screamadelica, **Primal Scream**

It sounds like a recipe for disaster. A failing retro-rock band, obsessed with leather trousers and '70s hair, were paired with a small-time club DJ for a B-side remix. With nothing to lose, he junked all of the song except for a fragment of bassline, rebuilt it from the ground up, and created a dancefloor monster: "Loaded." An album followed, which balanced euphoric dance tracks with traditional rock ballads, duly becoming the soundtrack to a generation's parties. It still sounds incredible today, with spacey wonderment, killer grooves, and, in "Don't Fight It, Feel It," a manifesto for all of us. "Ramalamalama, fa-fa-fa" sings Denise Johnson, "Gonna get high 'til the day I die." Well said.

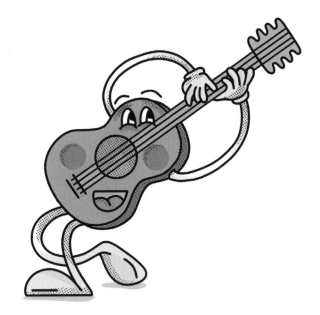

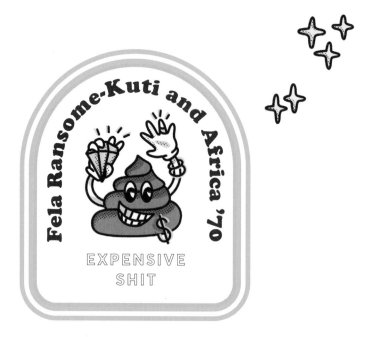

Expensive Shit, Fela Ransome-Kuti and Africa '70

The anarchic Afrobeat pioneer Fela Kuti was a huge star in '70s Nigeria, to the point that he could declare the compound where his family and bandmates lived an independent republic. For the ruling military junta, this was a provocation too far, and in one raid on the compound, the police planted a joint on him. Before he could be arrested and charged, Fela disposed of the evidence— by eating it—so the furious police locked him up until it emerged at the other end. Apparently Fela was able to procure another inmate's feces—the titular "expensive shit"—passed it off as his own, and was released. A great story, but still nothing like as good as the music on this two-track album: infectious brass and keyboard hooks punching out over Tony Allen's virtuosic drums. A classic.

Phoenix, The Warlocks

Showcasing stoner classics "The Dope Feels Good" and "Shake the Dope Out," this garage rock indie classic is full of guitars, tunes, and indie cool.

Black Messiah, D'Angelo

The sound of a major talent returning from a fourteen-year-long journey through the wilderness, *Black Messiah* is smoky, dense, deep, and rewarding.

Head Hunters, Herbie Hancock

Loping, repetitive, infectious, funky, melodic, rhythmic jazz funk. This is music to nod your head to while another bowl gets packed...

Paul's Boutique, Beastie Boys

No one expected the Beasties to come up with this. They were known for their brattish, juvenile raps, laid over hard-rock samples, and aimed at a predominantly white audience, but left to their own devices after the phenomenal success of their debut *Licensed to Ill*, they produced a sprawling masterpiece that dives deep into soul, funk, and disco for its grooves—while their earlier bellowed vocals are replaced (mostly) by looser, more rambling raps. It was a massive step forward, but it confused their audience, and completely bombed.

- BEASTIE BOYS -

PAUL'S B°UTIQUE

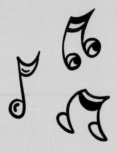

Ten Party Debuts

Here's a selection of albums that are great when the smokers come by and you need something uplifting, for more of a party vibe.

1 *Cypress Hill*, Cypress Hill
A smoking debut from this innovative West Coast crew, who went on to enjoy colossal success and a long and honorable career of weed advocacy.

2 *Bizarre Ride II the Pharcyde*, The Pharcyde
Another West Coast classic, with likable rhymes and grooves that are so laid-back as to be practically couchlocked.

3 *Supa Dupa Fly*, Missy Elliott
The title track alone makes this one a stoner's classic. Disconnected snippets of sound, a spacey, low-tempo groove, smoky inhalations and exhalations, and an impossibly composed delivery. And that's before you get to "Pass da Blunt"…

4 *Enter the Wu-Tang (36 Chambers)*, Wu-Tang Clan
The characteristically muffled, smoky sound of RZA's production has been credited to the early Akai samplers that he used to assemble the crew's grimy loops. Well, yes. That, or the weed. Shot through with black humor, this is full of hooks, classic beats, and memorable rhymes.

5

Avalanches, The Avalanches

An entire album patched together from hundreds of samples—many of those samples culled from frankly terrible easy-listening tunes—this is endlessly rewarding, filled with "moments" that weed-primed listeners love, and is danceable to boot.

6

Gorillaz, Gorillaz

Tunes, grooves, rhymes, hits, and a fully realized melting pot of rock, ska, hip-hop, and reggae. Pretty good, for a cartoon band made of fictional characters.

7

Show and Prove, Wiz Khalifa

Wiz has risen to become weed royalty, smoking staggering amounts and winning such a reputation on the scene that his endorsement can launch a new strain onto the market. His debut never sold as much as his later work, but it's among his best: easy on the ears, smooth, and full of simple grooves.

8

Nuyorican Soul, Nuyorican Soul

A timeless record, packed with fresh disco beats, soulful vocals, and jazzy licks from an all-star collection of talent. Latin to the core: one to follow a nice uplifting haze smoke.

9

Endtroducing, DJ Shadow

Another party album that's entirely cobbled together from tiny pieces of other albums, this is remorselessly groovy and dense with riffs, hooks, and beats upon beats.

10

Homework, Daft Punk

Squelching, melodic synths, banging house beats, and nonsensical lyrics, this deceptively minimal debut remains catchy as hell and is guaranteed to get you moving.

Ten Inner Flights

Otherwise known as music to chill by, these are perfect for when you're couchlocked by kush—just make sure you've got the remote at hand…

1 Electric Counterpoint, Steve Reich

Repetitive, pulsating textures that draw you in, suck you along, and show you sonic landscapes that you never knew existed. It's all guitar, but it doesn't sound like any guitars you've ever heard. Close your eyes and just get *bathed* in the waves of sound.

2 Blue Lines, Massive Attack

Astonishingly assured debut from a Bristol sound system, this was one of the earliest records to mash up reggae, hip-hop, and soul. To this day it still sounds fresh, atmospheric, and moving.

3 Yoshimi Battles the Pink Robots, Flaming Lips

A psychedelic alternative rock adventure that's packed with yearning tunes, lush production, and an underground unpredictability. The epic "Do You Realize?" is a highlight—the rare sound of a rock band seriously engaging with mortality. If you're in a poignant mood, it may all prove a little *too* emotional.

4 Dummy, Portishead

A mashup of film soundtracks, torch songs, and hip-hop breaks, this put Beth Gibbons' vulnerable, fragile vocals over minimal beats and atmospheric backing tracks. Feeling lonely? Feeling abandoned? A little paranoid? Try this. Beth understands how you feel, even if no one else does.

5
The Dark Side of the Moon, Pink Floyd
A staple of the stoner genre, this retains its capacity to surprise and transport nearly fifty years after its recording. Listen to this on the best stereo you can, get as high as you can, and be transported by the Floyd's inventiveness.

6
Grateful Dead ("Skull & Roses"), Grateful Dead
No list of stoner albums could be complete without a contribution from the Dead. This, their biggest seller, catches them live, in their pomp, showing off the harmonies, solos, and sense of adventure that made them the most abiding of all the freak bands.

7
Revolution Dub, Lee Perry & The Upsetters
Like the Grateful Dead, "Scratch" knew his way around a joint, and like them he was prolific, churning out dozens of classic dub sides from his Black Ark studio. This deep, sparse dub record is a highlight: drenched in echo, minimal grooves, and a unique sense of space.

8
On Fire, Galaxie 500
Repetitive, slow, lo-fi indie rock that draws you in and in with looping chord sequences, pleading vocals, and pulsating rhythms. Buried in it are some dreamy melodies and some killer guitar.

9
Masterpiece, Andrew Weatherall
Achieving near-divine status in his native UK, Weatherall was a remixer, producer, and dance DJ whose sound evolved continuously over his thirty-year career yet remained identifiably his. This collection of looping, down-tempo grooves is the perfect accompaniment to either a couchlock or a two-hour dance: a constant beat, overlaid with chunky baselines, occasional vocals, spacey percussion, and looping synths.

10
Ladies and Gentlemen We Are Floating in Space, Spiritualized
Not so much an album as a deep, deep dive into the area where doomed love affair meets hopeless drug addiction, this is a masterpiece of drugged-out gospel rock.

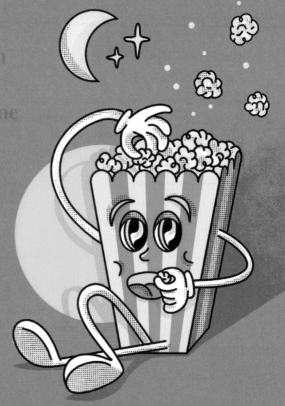

A Night at the Movies

Take a stoned brain on travels to places you never knew existed.

A reefer and the remote control bring new meaning to "Netflix and chill." Why sit in a sea of other people's popcorn at the movies when you can get comfy, roll up, and munch on whatever you please while watching a movie from the comfort of your own sofa? If you like, you can stretch out and enjoy a stoner comedy—but these are usually not great to watch, whether you're stoned or not. These usually feature a couple of amiable losers, struggling to complete simple tasks, or sentences—which grew out

Seek out richer, more sophisticated, mind-blowing experiences, for a more meaningful smoke.

of the '70s heyday of comic duo Cheech & Chong. Since the success of *Dude, Where's My Car?*, predictable re-treads have become a significant earner for Hollywood. Instead, you could seek out richer, more sophisticated, mind-blowing experiences, for a more meaningful smoke. How about a mind-bending sci-fi that will explore all your perceptions of space while you're spaced, or be inspired by a movie with a soundtrack to stir the soul, or try to navigate your way through a plotline that will make you question just how much you've had. Here's a list of some favorite movies to watch with marijuana; some are classics, some might be a bit more of a surprise, but none require more effort than simply getting to the sofa.

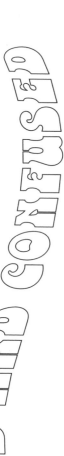

Dazed and Confused, dir. Richard Linklater (1993)

A hymn to the '70s, the suburbs, and high school, this classic coming-of-age comedy follows the progress of several groups of teenagers as they negotiate the last day of school in 1976. The high-schoolers victimize the middle-schoolers, the girls and boys circle each other with varying degrees of awkwardness, and there is pot *everywhere*. Adults—apart from a pair of ludicrous football coaches—are conspicuous by their absence: it's all about the interactions of the kids as they bounce around the Austin suburbs like the balls on a pool table. Even when they're being horrible to each other, Linklater's characters remain (mostly) sympathetic: nearly all of them are likable, awkward, lacking confidence—all too human—and the movie is packed with classic rock tracks and weed-friendly laughs.

Apocalypse Now, dir. Francis Ford Coppola (1979)

The last U.S. service personnel were pulled out of Vietnam in April 1975. Less than a year later, Francis Ford Coppola was on the ground in the Philippines, preparing to shoot what would come to be not only one of the defining cinematic visions of the Vietnam War, but one of the defining cinematic visions of war, full stop. Members of the cast were out of control: Martin Sheen drank himself to the point of heart attack, Dennis Hopper tormented everyone, and Marlon Brando refused to learn his lines. The movie ran hugely over budget and took years to produce; Coppola was driven to the brink, financially and psychologically. Yet out of this mess, miraculously, emerged a movie that was violent, beautiful, intelligent, horrifying, and intense. Best watched on a big screen as a happy brownie kicks in, *Apocalypse Now* is packed with *whoa!* moments, as Sheen's Captain Willard sails upriver, through the threatening jungle, toward a fatal confrontation with Brando's mysterious Kurtz.

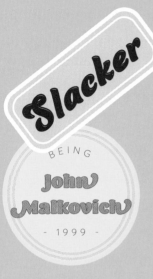

Slacker, dir. Richard Linklater (1990)

A low-budget guerilla production with no plot and no stars, Linklater's first feature is made arresting by its compelling portrait of alternative life in Austin. His characters drift from encounter to encounter: no one stays around for more than a few minutes before the baton is passed to another set of drifters for another inconsequential conversation. Ask yourself if his characters are heroic in their rejection of straight society—or just losers? A good one to watch on a sunny weekday morning, when you really should have something better to do, but it's hard to muster the energy…

Being John Malkovich, dir. Spike Jonze (1999)

An unpredictable, imaginative swing through a dazzling sequence of original ideas. What would it be like to find a portal into a movie star's head? To discover that you could control them like a puppet? To use them to seduce a co-worker? And how would it play out if several people started using the portal at once, each to their own ends…? Packed with wit, pitch-perfect performances, and sequences of stunning inventiveness, this will take a stoned brain to places you never knew existed.

Mad Max: Fury Road, dir. George Miller (2015)

A rare example of a remake completely trouncing its source material, this is possibly the purest action movie of all time: a crazy futuristic rampage through the desert with incredible vehicles and stunts, luminous cinematography, and dialogue that largely consists of grunts and screams. Tom Hardy, as Max, barely has a line to speak; the story is carried by Charlize Theron's Furiosa, a feminist freedom fighter. A rousing speed-fest that deserves a high audience, this won't challenge your brain, but it brings an undeniable rush.

The Harder They Come, dir. Perry Henzell (1972)

Reggae was the national music of Jamaica and had a small—if devoted—following in the U.K. Then *The Harder They Come* happened, and the world knew what it was, and where it had come from. Telling the story of Ivan, a struggling country boy who can sing but is driven into a life of crime, the movie not only realistically depicts Jamaican life (which made it a huge domestic hit) but also showcases songs that would define reggae for a global audience: "You Can Get It If You Really Want," "Pressure Drop," and the title number among them. Spark up a nice big spliff, get in a ganja frame of mind, and be grateful that you don't have to risk life and limb like Ivan does.

Inside Out, dir. Pete Docter (2015)

A Pixar movie? On this list? *Really?* Well, yes. If you're the kind of smoker who goes a little thoughtful and introverted when you're high, this is *exactly* the movie for you. Dramatizing the emotional life of a tween girl named Riley, this movie mostly takes place in her head, which, in Docter's vision, is a surreal technicolor landscape of control towers, vanishing islands, a gigantic memory store, and a surreal "train of thought" railroad. The sort of landscape, in fact, that a six-year-old can enjoy every bit as much as a stoned millennial. The lead characters are Riley's emotions: Joy, Sadness, Anger, Fear, and Disgust, and the surprisingly affecting storyline follows their struggles as she seeks to find happiness and balance. Believe me, you'll be tearing up at the end, even if you're not baked on hash brownies, which I recommend as a suitable accompaniment.

INSIDE OUT

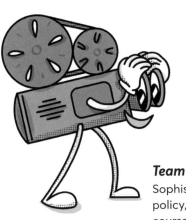

Team America: World Police, dir. Trey Parker (2004)

Sophisticated, ironic satire on the failures of U.S. foreign policy, or amateurish, juvenile gag-fest? The answer, of course, is both. Retaining their anarchic, irreverent humor, the *South Park* team dropped their usual lo-fi animation in favor of puppetry, with gloriously offensive results. Strings visible at all times, the calamitously stupid members of Team America shoot their way around the world in a quest to "save the motherfuckin' day, yeah" from Islamist terrorists, Kim Jong-Il, and left-wing, bleeding-heart, liberal Hollywood stars. Along the way, two characters, in a cinematic *tour de force*, have mind-blowingly hot sex. This suits group watching, passing the bong around, and group hilarity.

Withnail & I, dir. Bruce Robinson (1987)

London, the end of the 1960s. A pair of struggling actors decide to leave their disgusting flat and take a vacation: as they drink and drug themselves stupid, their relationship tragically, hilariously, comes apart at the seams. With career-defining performances from both its leads, *Withnail & I* earns its place on this list thanks to the immortal scene in which Danny the dealer drops by; "The joint I am about to roll," he tells them, "can utilize up to twelve skins. It is called the Camberwell Carrot..." An inspiration to architecturally minded smokers ever since, Danny and his carrot have influenced the creation of many joints that were really much larger than they had to be...

mulholland drive

Mulholland Drive, dir. David Lynch (2001)

A mysterious exploration of a dream-like Hollywood, this opens with a simple mystery: a struggling actress tries to help a car-crash victim remember her identity. At the same time, mobsters menace a film director, and a hitman looks for a book of phone numbers. The connections between all of the characters are unclear, and nothing seems to make sense—until a huge twist about four-fifths of the way through, after which… well, nothing makes much sense then, either. But it is enticing and lyrically shot, with excellent performances—particularly from the pair of female leads—and a seductive air of uncertainty and doubt. You'll want to talk this one through afterward, so don't overdo the weed!

Shaun of the Dead, dir. Edgar Wright (2004)

All of the great zombie movies are cut through with humor—it's a fundamentally ridiculous concept, after all—but *Shaun of the Dead* is possibly the funniest of them all. Against the backdrop of a zombie invasion of London, Shaun (Simon Pegg) does his best to shepherd his loved ones (and some of his less-loved ones, too) to safety. Bickering throughout, his party of survivors finally find shelter in the local pub—where the climactic showdown, cut to Queen's "Don't Stop Me Now"—reveals them to be spectacularly inept zombie killers. The relatable love story gives this movie plenty of heart, making it a great watch for a couple, particularly a couple who find it hard to get off the sofa and actually do something interesting…

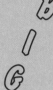
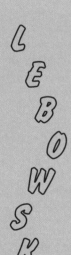

The Big Lebowski, dir. Coen Brothers (1998)

Now universally recognized as the finest stoner movie of its time, and one of the finest Hollywood movies of the '90s, *The Big Lebowski* was given mixed reviews on its release and was not a box office hit. Over time, though, its virtues became clearer, with midnight screenings, fan conferences, and numerous academic texts testifying to its power. Two African spider species have even been named for it (*Anelosimus dude* and *Anelosimus biglebowski*). The secret of the movie's success is that its hero, the Dude, offers not just snappy one-liners, but an aspirational lifestyle and philosophy package. A little tai chi, a little bowling, the occasional acid flashback, the occasional white Russian—and plenty of joints. All you need for a long, happy, productive life, right?

The Blues Brothers, dir. John Landis (1980)

One of the strangest movies ever made, a hybrid that lurches like a beat-up police cruiser from comedy sketch to musical showstopper to stunt-driving sequence and back again. There is a plot, but it's nothing but an excuse to connect National Lampoon-style skits to classic songs belted out by America's best singers and musicians. The soundtrack—Aretha! Ray! James!—is sensational throughout; the comedy has dated a little; the car chases remain hilariously pointless. Invite over a couple of close friends (the ones who you know like *good* music), pre-roll your joints so you've always got one ready to fire up, then crank up the volume. Don't ask yourself how this crazy edifice got signed off, just be grateful that it did.

Fight Club, dir. David Fincher (1999)

Hinging on one of the greatest onscreen plot reveals ever, *Fight Club* faces off Edward Norton's dweeby insurance assessor against Brad Pitt's provocative soap salesman. Where one is a conventional, consumer-oriented, white-collar worker, the other is a bare-knuckle fighter who asks "How much can you know of yourself if you've never been in a fight?"—justifying his violent urges with a seductive anticapitalist message. Appealing to the anarchist lurking inside all of us, the movie raises the stakes until the two leads arrive at a climactic face-off. Smoke your joint, and ask yourself: how committed are *you* to smashing the system?

The Matrix, dir. the Wachowskis (1999)

Many sci-fi movies claim to engage with philosophical ideas, but few do so as coherently and dramatically as *The Matrix*. A fundamental question of existence drives the action here, with Keanu Reeves' Neo joining a motley crew of freedom fighters struggling to break the power of the titular matrix—a software simulation that has trapped humanity. Reeves is great, and so is Carrie-Anne Moss as Trinity, but the show is stolen by Laurence Fishburne, who exudes a cool authority as Morpheus, expositor-in-chief, and Hugo Weaving, as the chilling Agent Smith. The special effects have dated a little; the sunglasses have dated a lot. The movie remains compelling, though, and is sure to prompt philosophical discussions afterward. Would *you* take the red pill?

Memento, dir. Christopher Nolan (2000)

Nolan's first movie, and probably his best—especially if you're busy adjusting your perceptions with a blunt as it runs. It tells the bewildering story of Leonard (Guy Pearce)

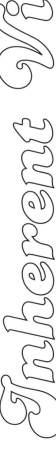

from two narratives, intercut, and running backward and forward toward the same point. Leonard has a form of amnesia that means he can't form short-term memories, making the world a confusing place full of people not to be trusted. Confusing? Yes. Gripping? Absolutely. Hard to follow when you're high? Mmmm-hmmm. And in case you're wondering, the movie's depictions of memory damage are, according to medical professionals, among the most realistic ever committed to film.

Be Kind Rewind, dir. Michel Gondry (2008)

One of the best things about marijuana is the way it bonds us, bringing us together with happy rituals of sharing, friendship, and togetherness. *Be Kind Rewind* doesn't have a single whiff of herb in it, but it's dank with community spirit and brotherly love. In a low-rent corner of New Jersey, Mike (Mos Def) and Jerry (Jack Black) are left in charge of a declining video store. They manage to destroy the stock, and in their efforts to rescue the business accidentally reinvent the art of cinema—and bring the town together. With all Gondry's trademark visual inventiveness, a ton of sight gags, and a heartwarming ending, this is a movie that celebrates the bonds we share.

Inherent Vice, dir. P.T. Anderson (2014)

Every ten years or so we get a fresh take on the L.A. private-detective noir genre, and *Inherent Vice* is a worthy addition to the canon. Joaquin Phoenix gives a great performance as the hippy detective, Doc, and the action follows him around an L.A. where—of course—the police are brutal, the women are alluring, and no one is to be trusted. The plot is convoluted, as it should be: there's slapstick humor, there's weirdness, and once it's finished, you'll probably want to start it right over again.

Five Movies Made for Stoners...

Let's be honest: most movies made for stoned audiences are pretty lame. Just because you're baked doesn't mean you're stupid, right? Sometimes, though, they hit the spot. Here are five films that take the clichés of stoner movies and put them to good use.

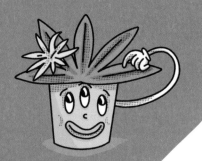

1

Cheech & Chong's *Up in Smoke*, dir. Lou Adler (1978)

Establishing all of the stoner genre's key clichés, *Up in Smoke* probably had a greater influence on Hollywood than its comedy really merits. Two guys, driving around in a car, meeting hot girls, trying to pull off the big score, and accidentally feeding drugs to a dog… it's all here, and nearly every line of dialogue ends "… man" to boot. Still, it makes for excellent stoned viewing.

2

Fast Times at Ridgemont High, dir. Amy Heckerling (1982)

There was always one guy at school who loved to smoke a little too much, right…? At Ridgemont High, that guy is Jeff Spicoli, a likable yet feckless, deep-tanned surf dude played with utter conviction by Sean Penn. A stellar ensemble cast (this movie kick-started not only Penn's career, but those of Jennifer Jason Leigh, Judge Reinhold, Eric Stoltz, Forest Whitaker, and Phoebe Cates) bring Ridgemont High to glorious life, with a little love, a little sex, a little sport, and history lessons from time to time, too. If possible, watch this one in a hot box, to faithfully replicate the atmosphere of a VW camper van full of pot smoke.

3

True Romance, dir. Tony Scott (1993)

It's a very simple love story, really. Boy meets girl, boy marries girl, boy kills pimp and accidentally steals a huge amount of mob cocaine, sparking a delirious road trip that's violent, fast-paced, slick, and, yes, romantic too. Christian Slater and Patricia Arquette turn in career-best performances, the supporting cast is stellar, and Tony Scott's direction is slick. The screenplay—an early piece of work by one Quentin Tarantino—is packed with the wisecracking menace that we've come to expect from his dialogue. But what makes it a stoner movie? Brad Pitt's immortal turn as the useless pothead Floyd, who plays a key role in the action while barely making it off the couch.

4

Harold & Kumar Go to White Castle, dir. Danny Leiner (2004)

The setup is a familiar one. Two stoners get the munchies and head to a burger joint, but this is a stoner comedy, so obviously things won't go according to plan. They duly don't, and the amiable heroes experience the usual misadventures: mistaken identity, celebrity cameo, friendly strippers, angry animals, beautiful neighbors, inept cops, white supremacists, and all. What lifts it above the run of the mill is the movie's stereotype-busting approach to race (Harold is Korean-American, Kumar is Indian-American) and the warmth of their friendship.

5

South Park: Bigger, Longer & Uncut, dir. Trey Parker (1999)

The characters are the same, the animation remains sketchy and low budget, and the stroke of genius of this movie-take on the long-running adult cartoon was making it a musical. The songs—conventional Broadway-style arrangements—are packed with filth, from the brilliantly abusive "Uncle Fucka" to "Blame Canada" or "Kyle's Mom's a Bitch." It's guaranteed to crack you up, even if you're not already plenty high, which you should be. The plot's ludicrous, of course: the U.S. and Canada go to war, causing Satan to rise up from hell, but that's not the point.

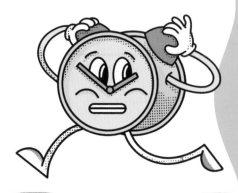

Five Time-Travel Mind-Benders

Perfect mind-twisters when you're twisting your mind—sit back, light up, and try not to think too hard…

1 *12 Monkeys*, dir. Terry Gilliam (1995)

Sent back from the future in order to prevent a viral outbreak destroying civilization, Cole (Bruce Willis) discovers his best lead in a psychiatric hospital, where the deranged environmentalist Goines (Brad Pitt, in full spider-chewing mode) is incarcerated. Repeated trips back and forward in time (the machine that sends him is wildly unreliable) slowly reveal the source of the virus, with a series of twists right up to the very last line of the movie.

2 *Primer*, dir. Shane Carruth (2004)

The lowest-budget movie on this list, and one of the most ingenious, *Primer* shows how time travel isn't just paradoxical: it's *incredibly* messy. Two engineers accidentally invent a box that allows them to travel back in time: initially careful about the consequences, they soon lose control, and multiple versions of themselves from different timelines end up fighting each other, bending reality, and blowing your mind.

3

Eternal Sunshine of the Spotless Mind, dir. Michel Gondry (2004)

Not strictly speaking a time-travel movie, this does deal in alternate realities and has a good chunk of pseudo-science driving the plot, so we can give it a pass. Joel (Jim Carrey) and Christine (Kate Winslet) meet on a train and immediately form a bond: it transpires that they're not meeting for the first time. Gondry's usual visual tricks fill the movie with arresting moments and the performances throughout are excellent.

4

Donnie Darko, dir. Richard Kelly (2001)

One for the troubled and directionless among us, this study in alienation follows Donnie (Jake Gyllenhaal), a teenager who is troubled by visions of Frank, a man in a bunny suit. Over the month of October, Donnie, guided by Frank, creates havoc in his small town—or does he?

5

Groundhog Day, dir. Harold Ramis (1993)

Forced to rerun the most boring, frustrating day of his life, TV weatherman Phil (Bill Murray) is stuck in a time loop: granted immortality, he is too immature to take advantage of it. Light, heartwarming, sentimental, this is a wholesome treat to share with a loved one and a mild, calming smoke.

Five Weird Visions

Some movies are very hard to unsee. This collection has more than its fair share of grotesque, hallucinatory visions; populated by memorable creatures, they are guaranteed to give an altered consciousness plenty of material to work with...

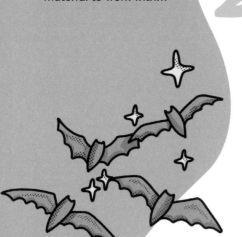

1 Pan's Labyrinth, dir. Guillermo del Toro (2006)

Setting a powerful fairy tale in the brutal context of Spain's civil war, this moving story of innocence struggling against oppression becomes classic stoner viewing by the fantastical character designs and supernatural settings. We follow the girl Ofelia (Ivana Baquero) as she is brutalized by her new stepfather, challenged by mysterious creatures from the underworld, and surrounded by tragedy. Visually unforgettable, but terrifying, gripping, and moving too.

2 Fear and Loathing in Las Vegas, dir. Terry Gilliam (1998)

Over-the-top acting, over-the-top-cinematography, and a story that consists of little more than escalating drug abuse... what's not to like? Under the influence of Johnny Depp's vivid Hunter S. Thompson impersonation, the pulsating soundtrack, and a lurid late-'60s production design, you'll almost believe that you were with him on this epic bender yourself. Bad, yet horribly charismatic, behavior from beginning to end, and a fantastic ride when you really want to push the boundaries and smoke a little bit more than perhaps is wise.

Naked Lunch, dir. David Cronenberg (1991)

Freely adapted both from William Burroughs' book of the same name, and the events surrounding its writing, this is a grim journey through a world of talking insects, telepathic conversation, paranoia, and violence. Heroin-addicted Bill (Peter Weller) is an unshockable and understated protagonist, becoming strangely sympathetic as the movie goes on.

Alice in Wonderland, dir. Tim Burton (2010)

Mashing up the plots of both original *Alice* books, and stirring in elements of the rest of Lewis Carroll's surreal oeuvre, Burton goes all in with a ridiculous assault on the eyes and ears. Don't worry about the plot, just soak in the vision: lurid colors, warped faces, gravity-defying motion. Probably best enjoyed with some edibles on hand. Go on, take the extra brownie…

Avatar, dir. James Cameron (2009)

Given an effectively infinite budget after the success of *Titanic*, James Cameron spent a fortune creating a virtual world—Pandora—populated by luridly colored and weirdly animated aliens. The humans (hungry to mine the planet and destroy its ecosystem) are the bad guys; the aliens, in tune with nature, the goodies. It is incredibly silly, but kind of works if you loosen yourself up a little first…

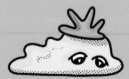

Five Rides into Paranoia

Too much weed makes you paranoid. I can't tell you anything more, because they're watching me. Just check these out. But don't tell anyone I told you.

1 ***Pi*, dir. Darren Aronofsky (1998)**

The secret of the universe is a 216-digit number. But don't let God know that you know.

2 ***The Conversation*, dir. Francis Ford Coppola (1974)**

Listening in to other people's conversations is a bad idea. What if they listen in on yours?

3 ***The Shining*, dir. Stanley Kubrick (1980)**

Don't work too hard. It may take its toll on your family life.

4 ***Contagion*, dir. Steven Soderbergh (2011)**

What if an invisible, unstoppable animal virus made it into the human population? What would happen then? Oh, *shit*.

5 ***The Wicker Man*, dir. Robin Hardy (1973)**

A pleasant rural island, with a law-abiding population. Such a lovely place to bring up a child.

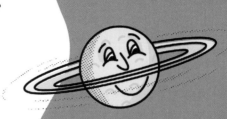

Nearly all space-travel movies require you to forget most of what you learned in science class: thanks to the weed, you're halfway there already.

1 *2001: A Space Odyssey*, dir. Stanley Kubrick (1968)

Where we came from, where we're going… it's a trip.

2 *Moon*, dir. Duncan Jones (2009)

You're the only man on the moon. Aren't you?

3 *Sunshine*, dir. Danny Boyle (2007)

The sun's stopped working. We need to change the batteries.

4 *Interstellar*, dir. Christopher Nolan (2014)

The world's stopped working. Let's move off.

5 *Gravity*, dir. Alfonso Cuarón (2013)

The capsule's stopped working. Let's learn Russian.

Get
Couchlocked

TV

You could turn your smoking session into something really rewarding.

OK, I know what you're thinking. It doesn't take much energy or creativity to get couchlocked, reach for the remote, and watch TV on your lonesome, does it? Well, possibly not. You could choose to chill out and binge-watch an unchallenging generic TV drama, or work your way through one network's evening schedule without thinking of changing the channel in an effort to wind down after a stressful day, or just to relax with your other half.

Or you could turn your smoking session into something really mentally rewarding or uplifting, perhaps even watching something with a few friends and getting a viewing party going. In the following pages you'll find a host of particularly rewarding TV experiences that offer a little something extra, and, in many cases, are eye-opening. Whether it's a deep, mysterious drama, a rather riotous comedy, an informative documentary, or just a good old simple animation (for kids or adults—whatever's your guilty pleasure!), each selection here is a tender bud, just waiting for you to sit back and enjoy it.

Whether it's a deep, mysterious drama, a particularly riotous comedy, or an informative documentary, each selection here is a tender bud, just waiting for you to enjoy it.

Drama

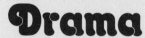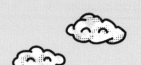

TV to stay awake to. For those nights when you want
a civilized toke and some quality viewing.

Russian Doll

Ever get the feeling that you're stuck in a loop? Ever get
the feeling that the drugs might not be quite as much fun
as they seem? Ever fallen down the stairs? *Russian Doll* is
for you: a dizzyingly inventive riff on *Groundhog Day* that
takes a hip Manhattan birthday party as its starting point
and gradually unfolds layer after mysterious layer on its
way to a surprisingly uplifting denouement.

Angels in America

It's impossible to disentangle the medical marijuana
movement from the early years of the HIV/AIDS crisis,
and this visionary realization of Tony Kushner's stage play
brings that moment of crisis, fear, and denial vividly to life.
It's not, though, a realistic drama, but a visionary one:
the suffering leads are visited by angels and ghosts—
watch this when you are ready for some really
extraordinary viewing.

Weeds

Well, this one really *had* to be in here. Back in 2005, when
it first aired, a mom who started selling weed to fund her
family's lifestyle was a criminal—and in due course, she
had to go on the run to stay free. These days, you'd call
her a cannapreneur, or a mompreneur, and she'd move
down the road to a bigger house.

Kidding

Imagine a cross between *Mister Rogers' Neighborhood* and *Sesame Street* created by a loving, caring, yet deeply dysfunctional family. That's the setup: Jim Carrey is Mr. Pickles, around whose sincere, caring presence director Michel Gondry orchestrates a drama of lies, grief, and a little bit of weed. The border between Mr. Pickles' reality and the action of his children's show blurs, yielding a string of surreal reveals, and this show takes some surprising routes to emotional and psychological depths.

Lost

A plane crash. A mysterious island. Good-looking survivors with intriguing character flaws and tragic backstories. A polar bear in the jungle. A monster made of smoke. Nonsense, really, but it will suck you in and spark theorizing conversations that will seem *very important* at the time.

RuPaul's Drag Race

Emotion! Drama! Artificial fibers! Year after fabulous year, *RuPaul's Drag Race* erupts onto our screens like a heartfelt, colorful blob of pure bitchiness. The contest drives increasingly desperate, incredibly talented, wildly vulnerable drag queens through a series of drag challenges: the bitchy put-downs come thick and fast, but there's always a moment of feelgood affirmation to get the tears coming, too.

Black Mirror

A horribly inventive series of standalone dramas that take our dependence on technology as a starting point and spin it off into sinister directions. Twisty, dark, cynical, with a pessimistic view of human nature and microprocessors alike, these shows will leave you staring with paranoid suspicion at your phone. What's *in* there...?

The X-Files

If you were a conspiracy theorist in the 1990s, this was your go-to show. Over 200 episodes pitted two FBI agents against a wide array of supernatural and extraterrestrial foes: over time, Mulder and Scully uncover a secret plot to take over the world by... no, wait. I won't spoil it for you. One part anti-institutional paranoia to two parts monster-of-the-week, this remains excellent viewing.

Star Trek

The original *Star Trek* hasn't lost anything in the fifty years since it first transmitted. The costumes are still amazing, the plot setups surprisingly thought-provoking, and the special effects are... well, they're good enough, if you're high. A toke or two will help you enjoy the hidden philosophical subtexts. Later iterations of the series gained in visual impact and production values, but maybe lost some of the charm that makes the original such compelling viewing for the high among us...

Comedy

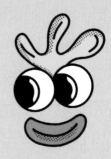

Sometimes you just need to get high and watch something that really doesn't challenge you on any level at all. These are shows that you can fall asleep to, wake up ten minutes later, and know that you won't have any trouble catching up...

Mystery Science Theater 3000

Feeling lonely? Want to just kick back and watch some TV with friends, but there's nobody around? Never fear, *MST3K* is here to help. Join Joel the janitor and his two robot buddies, Tom Servo and Crow T. Robot, as they talk over some of the worst movies ever made. Riffing on stilted dialogue and terrible special effects is more fun than you'd think. After a while, it's almost as if you're not alone any more...

Portlandia

In this life, you've got to be able to laugh at yourself. And if you're anywhere on the hipster-counterculture spectrum, you need to be laughing at *Portlandia*. Because it *nails* you. Us.

What We Do in the Shadows

Another comedy setup featuring flawed personalities trapped in insufficient space, this follows a quartet of out-of-place vampires and their human servant. The horror elements give this a gothic coating, but the most chilling is the energy vampire, Colin Robinson, who drains the spirits of his cubicle-farm coworkers in a way that's horribly relatable...

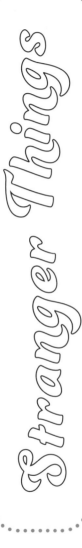
Stranger Things

Jackass

Something for the teenage boy in all of us, *Jackass* features a gang of self-destructive, tasteless, lowest-common-denominator pranksters doing terrible things to their own and each other's bodies in the name of a cheap laugh. Those cheap laughs do come, though, relentlessly. A terrifying glimpse into the American psyche: very stupid, and very, very funny.

Stranger Things

OK, this ran out of steam quite badly after the first couple of seasons, but its initial impact was huge and it makes perfect stoner viewing for so many reasons. There's the loving evocation of adolescent friendships and the stirrings of love. There's the sharp-as-a-tack '80s nostalgia, the killer performances from the entire cast, the genuine sense of peril and fear as we learn more about what threatens the town of Hawkins... hell, it even made *Dungeons & Dragons* cool again.

Sex Education

A 100 percent woke guide to twenty-first-century sexuality, this warm-hearted series is set in a bizarre hybrid of the U.K. and U.S., where a vividly colorful high school entertains love and sex in all its many forms. The uniformly excellent cast (mostly in their mid-twenties and playing characters that are much younger) bounce off each other in increasingly convoluted triangles and, like clockwork, make discoveries about how sex works as they do. Watch this with someone with whom you would like to move out of the friend zone, if you suspect that they might like to move out of the friend zone, too...

Documentaries

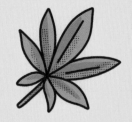

Is your mind open to wonder, to amazement, and maybe a little education? Try drifting along to one of these…

Cannabis: A Lost History

Educate yourself, without ever losing sight of your spliff. This gently paced documentary takes in the history of the herb from prehistoric times through classical civilization, up to prohibition and recent decriminalization. This flick will give you all manner of "did you know?" conversation gambits.

Grass is Greener

Fab Five Freddy, hip-hop pioneer and long-time weed advocate, tells the fascinating tale of cannabis's many connections with black music. Top-drawer interviewees and a long historical lens make this essential viewing, particularly when it comes to understanding the deep well of racism and prejudice that inspired prohibition back in the 1930s and 1940s.

The Culture High

Taking apart the war on drugs and telling the story of its progression from the 1970s to the twenty-first century, this film attacks the injustice of federal prohibition and is an eye-opening watch.

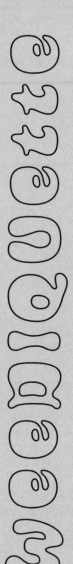

Super High Me

Doug Benson really likes weed, and in an effort to discover what it was doing to his body, went on a thirty-day smoking jag. At the end of it, he went through a series of medical and intellectual tests in order to measure the effect on his body and mind—which we won't spoil here—but they are worth the wait.

Weediquette

A Vice TV documentary strand that sees Krishna Andavolu looking for the most interesting stories in the world of weed—and finding them.

The Future of Weed: High Country

Another dive into the Colorado experience, this time from a business point of view, looking at how entrepreneurs seized the moment, making money—or losing it—and employing fascinating new techniques and technologies to maximize their returns.

Dimebags vs. Dispensaries

A special from Vice TV, this follows a pair of entrepreneurs as they transition from illegal to legitimate weed-dealing. It is useful viewing for anyone starting up a new business. The show also unpacks many facets of the legal cannabis business, including criminalization, racial inequality, and financial gain.

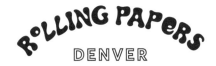

DENVER

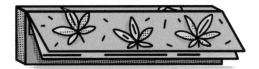

Rolling Papers

Weed changed Denver, and these changes needed reporting on, so the *Denver Post* appointed a Marijuana Editor to find those stories and cover them. This fascinating documentary reveals many of the surprising ways in which urban life can be changed by legalization.

Weed the People

If you're not suffering from serious illness yourself, the whole medical marijuana issue can seem a bit remote. It won't be once you've watched this moving introduction to the struggles of cancer patients who rely on the drug to relieve their symptoms—and the forces of prohibition aligned against them.

Breaking Habits

The number one cash crop in California is marijuana, and when your harvest is worth a cool $250K, it becomes a target for the bad guys—which makes you a target for the bad guys, too. The subjects of this doc are unique, such as the superfluity of feminist nuns on a mission to supply medical marijuana, who are not afraid to tote their own firearms to defend their crop. Yes, you read that right. Feminist marijuana nuns with guns. And yes, it's a documentary.

Bong Appétit

Bong Appétit

Cooking TV is fantastic TV, period. And cooking with cannabis is also fantastic. So it stands to reason that a cooking with cannabis TV show will also be good, and *Bong Appétit*—awful title aside—does not disappoint. ou'll pick up some cooking tips, as well as random nuggets of marijuana lore.

The Profit: Marijuana Millions

Watch this if you are wildly enthusiastic about the ways in which venture capital is changing the marijuana marketplace. In fact, watch it if you're not: you should really know how it works, in any case…

Cosmos

Forget about the remake: everything about the original *Cosmos*—the Carl Sagan version, from 1980—is television perfection, especially if you're blunted to the point of near-coma. The low-budget, pixelated visuals, the epic synthesizers, Sagan's reassuringly knowledgeable voice… it's all great stuff. The science may be a bit dated, but it's *definitely* educational.

The Blue Planet I & II

David Attenborough's classic run of high-concept nature documentaries might just have peaked with these two series. It turns out that the seas are full of more incredible sights than you ever expected: angler fish, fangtooths, and squid bring the weird; whales, dolphins, and clownfish are lovable; huge schools of herring, anchovy, and mackerel provide food for the more interesting stars of the show. Never has the soft gurgle of a bong been a more appropriate soundtrack.

Our Planet

Another nature show, and equally amazing. Dancing birds, jumping whales, tragic walruses... there isn't an emotion that won't be touched by these astonishingly filmed vignettes, each species given its own drama. Underpinning it all: a coherent, consistent message about the urgency of climate change.

Our Planet

The Joy of Painting (Bob Ross)

A stoner favorite for decades, Bob Ross's gentle, relentlessly positive creativity charms in every shade from titanium white to mountain-mixture gray. Bob doesn't judge you for getting high and spending hours on the couch watching back-to-back episodes of him dabbing Alaskan peaks, sociable trees, or happy little clouds. He just wants you to pursue your interests so they become talents. And if you ever make mistakes? "Let's make them birds. Yeah, they're birds now."

Slow TV: Train Ride Bergen to Oslo

Trains run from Bergen to Oslo four times a day, and the journey along a single-track line takes seven hours. The scenery is spectacularly beautiful: the railroad loops up into the mountains of central Norway, taking in meadows, forests, frozen lakes, and spectacular fjords on the way; a chilled landscape, especially in winter. You can enjoy the whole experience from the comfort of your den: chow down on a couple of brownies and let the buzz run for a few hours while the tracks draw you ever onward, through the fir forests and into the center of the screen...

Joons to Joke to

There's something ridiculously comforting about skinning up and relaxing into the surreal world of an offbeat animation. When you're utterly relaxed and feeling in the mood for something wholesome, unchallenging, and reassuring, there's nothing better than stepping back into your childhood—and catching up on your Saturday morning viewing. Alternatively, when you're nicely buzzing and ready to giggle, there's nothing like checking in with the adult animations…

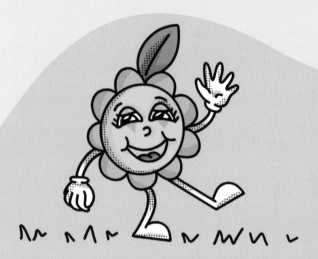

Futurama

Not *The Simpsons*, but every bit as funny and with an edge of desperation that never lets it get stale. Locked in a selection of dysfunctional relationships on the Planet Express Ship, the alien-human-robot crew don't just serve up classic workplace sitcom, but an astute skewering of the sci-fi genre, too.

Bob's Burgers

So very warm and wholesome, this is a slower burn and is perhaps suited to the long fade that comes some hours after a strong edible—there's no chance of the Belcher family's exploits triggering any anxiety or paranoia.

South Park

It's hard to imagine quite how shocking *South Park* was when it first dropped in the late '90s, with its sweary, young-boy protagonists, its cynical view of the state of American society, and its willingness to bust taboos left, right, and center. This heroic iconoclasm is what keeps it fresh: the show enthusiastically satirizes religion in particular, with the Church of Scientology, Mormonism, the Virgin Mary, and the Prophet Muhammad among its many sacrilegious depictions.

Rick and Morty

This one rewards total immersion. On the surface, it's sci-fi silliness, with time travel, laser beams, spaceships, and frequent gross-outs as unpleasant alien species dismember each other and, occasionally, the titular heroes. Dig down a little, and it irreverently raises a few big philosophical questions about the nature of time, and the implications of alternate realities. Down a little further, and it's a family drama, unpacking the complicated bonds between Morty, his disreputable grandfather Rick, his sister, and his mom and dad. At every level, the show generates laughs at a reliable pace. Smoke at the rate of one joint per episode, and binge-watch as far as you can…

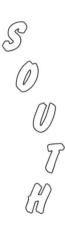

Archer

Ever dreamed that you worked in an office where everyone was exactly as rude as they wanted to be, all the time? *Archer* takes this uninhibited setup and applies it to a dysfunctional set of secret agents, with hilarious results. The early series in particular are rushes of wordplay, bitchiness, innuendo, camp, cynicism, and sexual perversity: the Cold War never looked so fun.

BoJack Horseman

The downside of Hollywood stardom is explored from, obviously, the perspective of a talking stallion. Join BoJack, an aging star with all kinds of psychological issues, as he lurches from embarrassment to disaster across a Tinseltown that's reimagined as an unlikely menagerie. Will he clean up? Will he find love? Will he always be tortured by remorse? You may be surprised to find yourself caring about the answers to all these questions, and forgetting that you're watching a cartoon horse. But, then, you are high.

Adventure Time

That rare thing—a toon that appeals equally to kids and adults—that doesn't need to draw on a constant stream of pop culture references to get by. Surreal, at times sad, this is childish in the best possible way.

SpongeBob SquarePants

Good-natured, heartwarming silliness as SpongeBob and his friends goof around the surreal landscape of Bikini Bottom. Man, it was *great* being a kid, wasn't it?

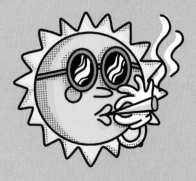

The Ren & Stimpy Show

How could this have been a kids' show? The characters are gross, ugly, and weird: Ren (the chihuahua) is horribly mean and aggressive to Stimpy (the cat), and there are often sinister undercurrents. Traumatizing a generation of Saturday morning toon-hounds before its cancellation (for unpunctuality, the most stoner-ish of reasons), *The Ren & Stimpy Show* is a simply magnificent accompaniment to a bong or a bucket.

The Simpsons

Of course, hundreds of episodes of *The Simpsons* are comedy gold for stoners, but the one that perhaps deserves your closest watch and deepest critical appreciation is episode sixteen of season thirteen—"Weekend at Burnsie's," during which Homer starts using medical marijuana perhaps a little more than his medical needs themselves would justify. The episode is notable for some particularly off-the-wall-moments (for no real reason, the family are menaced by crows, Smithers dresses as Judy Garland, and the band Phish make an appearance) and its nuanced take on Homer's experience. It's well worth a party watch, followed by an in-depth discussion of the issues raised, a critique of the animation's finer points, and another doobie.

The Emperor Wears No Clothes
The Cannabis Manifesto
The Pot Book
Cannabis for Couples
Ganja Yoga
Cannabis Climax
Marijuana Horticulture
A Beginner's Guide to
   Growing Marijuana
Feminist Weed Farmer
A Field Guide to
   Marijuana
Smoke Signals
Cannabis Pharmacy
A Woman's
   Guide to
   Cannabis
Exercises
   in Style
The Wild Party
On the Road
Wonder Boys
Chronic City
The Hasheesh Eater
Junky
Howard Marks' Book of Dope Stories
Artificial Paradises

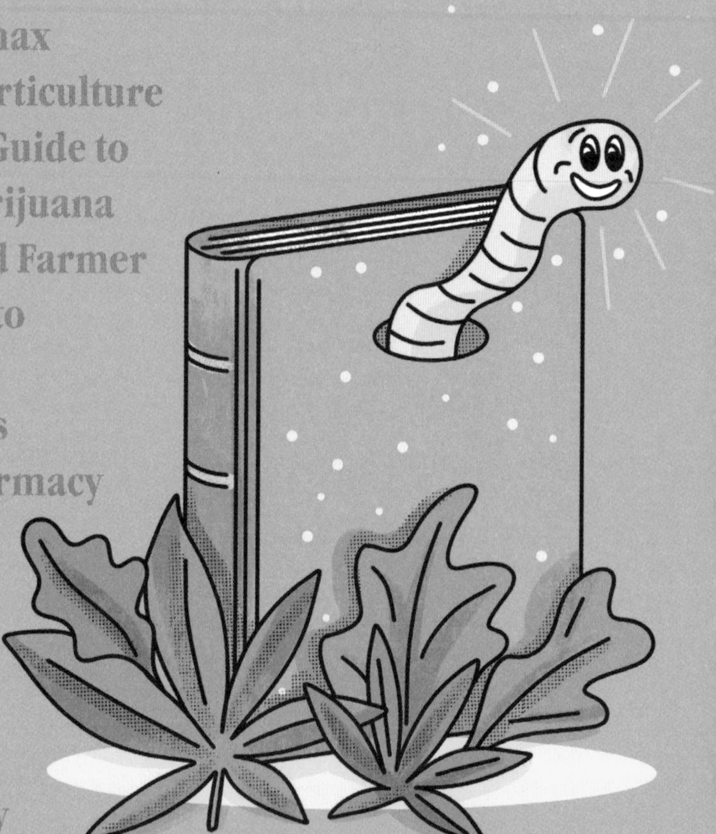

Books

If you pair your smoke and your reading material carefully, you can enjoy new perceptions and a particularly rich engagement with the written word.

No one expects you to partake of a heavy *indica* bud and then work your way through a tome like *War and Peace*, but if you pair your smoke and your reading material carefully, you can enjoy new perceptions and a particularly rich engagement with the written word. Apart from the obvious Beat and Gonzo classics, which remain excellent and highly relevant to the smoker, there's a host of great writing that you can enjoy with a reefer at hand—especially if you've picked a

No one expects you to partake of a heavy *indica* bud and then work your way through *War and Peace*.

stimulating *sativa* strain. From poetry to reportage, from spaced-out fiction to riveting stoner memoirs, there are books that will be educational in the history and finer points of toking, give a fascinating insight into the world of enigmatic master criminals, provide a literally "higher" level of reading to inspire you, as well as some that offer more cerebral topics for those deep and meaningful moments when you want to engage or reflect on life. So roll up and settle down with one of these suggestions, depending on your mood.

Informative Reads About the Weed

You should know what it is that you're smoking, why you like it so much, and what it can do for you and your world. Here are the fundamentals of cannaliterature for your education and entertainment.

The Emperor Wears No Clothes, by Jack Herer

This self-published volume, which has sold hundreds of thousands of copies and been updated and revised many times, was the first to lay out the argument for legalizing marijuana and letting it play a much larger part in the world economy. Herer's research reveals thousands of uses for hemp, from making cloth to biomass energy, and also tells its incredible history— and the sad tale of its prohibition. Read it for *huge* amounts of marijuana trivia, but also to inform yourself how we can use this miracle crop to make our planet a better place for everyone.

Edibles: Small Bites for the Modern Cannabis Kitchen, by Stephanie Hua and Coreen Carroll

Most of the time you want your edibles to be snackable, but a diet of brownies and cookies alone is unhealthy and monotonous. Pick up this popular volume if you want to broaden your repertoire with a range of sweet and savory bite-sized treats.

The Cannabis Manifesto: A New Paradigm for Wellness, by Steve DeAngelo

Taking a more focused look at cannabis's medical potential, this book by the world's leading cannabis entrepreneur will make you rethink everything you thought you knew about the subject, and it provides expert guidance on how to use it effectively. It's particularly revealing on how ineffective prohibition has been: when marijuana was banned in 1913, only 1 percent of the American population knew what it was—and one hundred years later, millions were breaking the law every day to enjoy it. Read this for expert insights into where weed came from, where it's going, and what it can do for you.

The Pot Book, edited by Julie Holland, M.D.

Presented more formally and authoritatively than *The Emperor Wears No Clothes*, this is now the standard single-volume guide to medical marijuana and the many therapeutic uses of CBD, THC, and the other cannabinoids, as well as including a wealth of other information. Each chapter is written by one of a team of specialists, most of whom are Ph.D.s or M.D.s. The book answers all your questions about the risks of vaporizers, the dangers of driving high, and the effects of prohibition, as well as the fine detail on how marijuana works its magic on the brain.

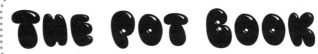

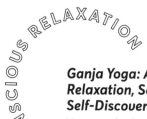

CONSCIOUS RELAXATION

Ganja Yoga: A Practical Guide to Conscious Relaxation, Soothing Pain Relief, and Enlightened Self-Discovery, by Dee Dussault

Yogis and other Asian mystics have been combining *bhang* with yoga and meditation for hundreds of years, but Dee Dussault was the first yoga teacher to carefully introduce conscious, intentional marijuana use into her practice in the U.S. This popular volume shows how you can do it yourself—with potentially profound results.

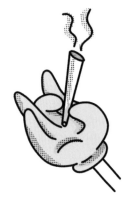

Cannabis Climax: The Connoisseur's Guide to Cannaphrodisiacs, by Bianca Latimer

You may be lucky enough to have explored this area already, but if you haven't, then let Latimer be your guide. She starts by looking at the ways that Indian mystics used *bhang* as part of their tantric sex practices, then goes on to explain and celebrate the many ways in which the weed can be useful for male and female lovers alike.

Marijuana Horticulture: The Indoor/Outdoor Medical Grower's Bible, by Jorge Cervantes

Ever wanted to grow your own? If you want to take your hobby to a horticultural—or agricultural—level, this grower's bible is what you need, covering everything from picking a strain to preparing your soil, choosing lights and ventilation systems… *everything*. The downside: at 500+ pages, this is not a light read, and its pages are densely packed with information. If you just want to grow a plant or two in the backyard, it may be a bit much…

Cannabis: A Beginner's Guide to Growing Marijuana, by Danny Danko

...so why not try this? Danny Danko is senior cultivation editor at *High Times* magazine, so he knows what he's talking about, and this is a punchy, simple guide that gets you up and running nice and fast. All of the key topics are covered, from genetics to pest control and harvesting, and Danko will take you to self-sufficiency with the minimum of effort.

Feminist Weed Farmer: Growing Mindful Medicine in Your Own Backyard, by Madrone Stewart

If you like your growing guides to be informative, friendly, and shot through with life lessons as well as growing tips, then this is for you: how to grow weed and grow as a person, in one package. Stewart's an expert on growing in general, and also has an entertaining turn of phrase ("if you find a male plant, kill it immediately") and plenty of thoughts on the encroaching corporatization of the scene.

Cannabis for Couples: Enhance Intimacy and Elevate Your Relationship, by John Selby

It's all very well to save the world by smoking weed, but can it also help your relationship? Seasoned relationship counselor John Selby lays out convincing arguments that intentional cannabis use can take your relationship to a deeper, more spiritual level. His ideas are backed up by brain research from the National Institute of Health and have a solid psychological and neurological underpinning; he also offers detailed advice on which strains to try under different circumstances.

Green: A Field Guide to Marijuana, by Dan Michaels and Erik Christiansen

If you're in the lucky position of being able to shop for your bud at a well-stocked dispensary, *Green* will be an invaluable guide through their stock and the bewildering range of buds now available. With over 150 different strains detailed, you'll be able to choose the perfect point on the *sativa–indica* spectrum for your needs, and the book also supplies (brief) tasting and smoking notes. The most distinctive aspect, though, is Christiansen's gorgeous photography: every bud is shot in close-up detail, giving you a mouthwatering preview of pistils, flowers, sugar leaves, and trichomes. If you're into growing your own, it doesn't offer much, but as a consumer's catalog, it's hard to beat.

Smoke Signals: A Social History of Marijuana, by Martin A. Lee

This might be the most readable of the standard histories of weed, opening with the memorable image of a cowboy policeman riding his horse to New York to make the argument for legalization, and closing with an inspiring, prophetic (the book came out in 2012) call to legalize.

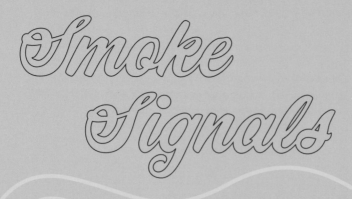

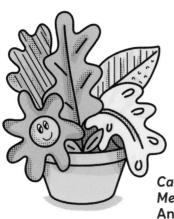

Cannabis Pharmacy: The Practical Guide to Medical Marijuana, by Michael Backes and Andrew Weil

If you want to start seriously informing yourself about marijuana's medical potential, this is a great place to start. There's a ton of evidence-based information on how to treat over fifty ailments, and an invaluable guide to the different strains and their varying effects—so you know when to dose with Banana Kush, and when with Kryptonite. There's advice on delivery and dosing, and a thorough breakdown of how the endocannabinoid system works. In 2007 Backes cofounded the Cornerstone Research Collective, the first evidence-based medical cannabis collective in California, and he is a prominent figure in cannabis research, so this is an authoritative, trustworthy source.

A Woman's Guide to Cannabis: Using Marijuana to Feel Better, Look Better, Sleep Better—and Get High Like a Lady, by Nikki Furrer

It was inevitable that, once cannabis's many benefits were properly identified, it would become a lifestyle product for those with more sophisticated aspirations than Cheech & Chong's—more specifically, for women. Nikki Furrer's handbook is an introduction to that way of life, and it's informative, fun, and packed with ways that any woman can improve her quality of life with just a little more marijuana.

Literary Explorers

Some writers, not necessarily big pot smokers themselves, experiment with their writing in a way that makes them irresistible to the higher reader.

Exercises in Style, by Raymond Queneau

The same simple story—about a brief altercation on a Parisian bus—told ninety-nine different ways, this is endlessly inventive and a fun introduction to applied literary theory. The versions are all very short, so stoned attention spans can cope, but the sheer joy and creativity make this a classic. You may, like many other readers, be inspired to write your own exercise.

The Wild Party, by Joseph Moncure March

Beloved of the Beats and all kinds of alternative authors, *The Wild Party* is an epic poem—but don't be put off if epic poems aren't usually your thing. This zings off the page and whips energetically through the fateful events of a too-hot New York night, as Queenie (a hard-drinking dancer) and her vicious lover Burrs (an even more hard-drinking clown) decide to throw a party. The whole thing is told in rhyming couplets, with the assertive, danceable rhythms of jazz driving events to their violent conclusion. Pick up the edition with illustrations by Art Spiegelman for a visual delight that matches the words.

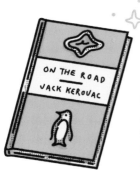

On the Road, by Jack Kerouac

Jack Kerouac was Canadian, and as a sailor he had traveled widely, but his greatest work is American through and through—a thinly disguised autobiographical collection of the adventures that he and his inspirational mentor Neal Cassady enjoyed on various road trips across the U.S. As Kerouac put it, it was "a journey through post-Whitman America to FIND that America and to FIND the inherent goodness in American man." Stylistically, it was radical, and it dealt freely with promiscuity, marijuana, jazz, and other hot topics. Read it if you want to know about the era when cannabis wasn't a common pursuit: when aggressive law enforcement, racism, and ignorance kept it underground, and when smoking a reefer—and writing about it—was a major statement of rebellion.

Wonder Boys, by Michael Chabon

We all know someone who smokes too much, has smoked too much for a very long time, and probably always will smoke too much. They behave badly, they let you down, and yet… they're still your friend. If that's a scenario you're familiar with, pick up *Wonder Boys*, in which one such character stumbles from one bad situation to the next.

Chronic City, by Jonathan Lethem

Surreal, multilayered, fanciful, and full of joints from beginning to end. Not for everyone (if you don't like novels with philosophical digressions and odd notes of fantasy in the realism, head for George Pelecanos instead) but entertaining, elegant, and clever all the same.

artificial paradises

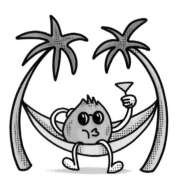

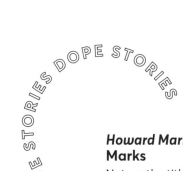

Howard Marks' Book of Dope Stories, by Howard Marks

Not, as the title would suggest, a series of anecdotes told by Howard Marks himself, but an anthology of writing about drugs (of all kinds) that he found interesting. He was widely read, had excellent taste, and knew his narcotics— so this is a terrific companion if you feel like dipping in for a shorter read and discovering a new writer.

Artificial Paradises, by Mike Jay

Another anthology, with a huge number of short reflections on any number of drug experiences, going as far back as Homer. Think of it as an alternative encyclopedia, full of insights, inspirations, and insobrieties.

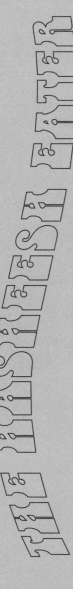

The Hasheesh Eater: Being Passages from the Life of a Pythagorean, by Fitz Hugh Ludlow

Ludlow was a young New Yorker who, in the middle of the nineteenth century, was prescribed cannabis to relieve the symptoms of lockjaw (tetanus). It's fair to say that he took more than the recommended dose and went spinning off on a visionary path that, like his contemporary Walt Whitman, inspired the Beats and hippies a century later.

The Road to Purification: Hustlers, Hassles & Hash, by Harry Whitewolf

The true story of Harry's low-key adventures as a dreadlocked stoner in and around Cairo, on a bender after the end of his relationship. We've all been there, but it's fair to say that most of us haven't taken heartbreak to quite such ludicrous and comical extremes as Harry has.

Junky, by William S. Burroughs

Like his friend Allen Ginsberg, Burroughs passionately believed in the creative power of weed. This book isn't specifically about that, but it's probably his most accessible, and is a courageous account of his life as a gay heroin addict in the conservative atmosphere of the 1950s.

Something Spiritual

If you're feeling receptive and free-floating thanks to that interesting *indica*, try something deep and meaningful.

The Prophet, by Kahlil Gibran

If you're of a spiritual, mystical turn of mind, then you will probably enjoy this much more than Thompson or Welsh. Gibran's collection of philosophical poems has sold millions of copies worldwide and continually speaks to new generations, notably, these days, poets like Rupi Kaur. The titular Prophet is the poet: he answers questions thrown at him by a crowd, with clear, elegant, sometimes paradoxical blank verse.

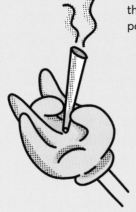

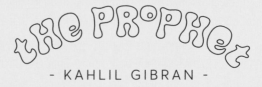

- KAHLIL GIBRAN -

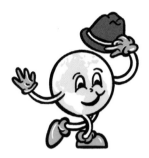

Pictures of the Gone World, by Lawrence Ferlinghetti

With Ginsberg, Ferlinghetti was the leading poet of the Beat movement, and also its key publisher. His work, though, is less agonized than his compatriot's. Ferlinghetti really loves life, and the key theme of his work is a desire that the human race finally live up to its beautiful potential. Check out "The World is a Beautiful Place," juxtaposing the joys of "making babies and wearing pants" with the horrors of "a bomb or two/now and then." A mellow high—the kind that gets you thinking warmly of other people, and enjoying the moment to its full potential—is an excellent accompaniment to Ferlinghetti's work.

Howl and Other Poems, by Allen Ginsberg

As noted elsewhere in this book, Allen Ginsberg was a keen smoker and advocate for weed; he was also America's leading poet of the 1950s and 1960s. *Howl* is the key work, and in it Ginsberg declares, "I smoke marijuana every chance I get." For him, it is one element of a profound rebellion against the stultifying conservatism of the postwar U.S.A., a nation that won't end the "human war." Much of it resonates today.

True Tales of Users and Dealers

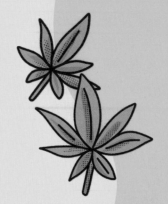

It's always fun to read a true tale of cops versus traffickers, or of pioneering potheads—even more so if you've got a nice *sativa* buzz on.

Mr. Nice, by Howard Marks

If you smoked hash in the 1970s and 1980s, there's a strong chance you had Howard Marks to thank for it. He ran a series of operations smuggling Nepalese, Thai, and Pakistani resin from Asia into the growing markets of Europe and North America, and in the mid-'70s he was flying tons at a time into John F. Kennedy airport. His business partners included such heavy organizations as the IRA, MI6, the Yakuza, the CIA, the Mob, the PLO, the Triads, and various Asian security forces, but Marks somehow made it through unscathed, and survived two jail terms—one in the U.K. and one in the U.S. *Mr. Nice* (named for one of Marks' many false names) is the book he wrote on release, a fast-moving tale of the trafficking life with laugh-out-loud stories and plenty of hard-earned life wisdom.

Narconomics, by Tom Wainwright

You wouldn't expect a writer from the *Economist* to produce one of the most revealing examinations of the world of cartels, bulk marijuana smugglers, and cocaine growers, but Wainwright's book is an informative ride through this dangerous territory. His conclusions are fascinating, too; by applying the logic of economics to the issues, and looking at cartels in the same way as business analysts look at "straight" corporations, he makes many surprising connections. It's entertaining to think of internationally feared drug lords suffering from the same problems as corporate middle managers. Along the way, he also makes a convincing argument for legalization. Read this if you're interested in the issues around that, and also if at any point you've been forced to source your weed illegally. This will tell you a lot about where it came from.

The Electric Kool-Aid Acid Test, by Tom Wolfe

Back to the 1960s, back to the counterculture, and back to the start of a new style of nonfiction writing. Ken Kesey's Merry Pranksters were the first prominent hippies: freaks who roamed the nation on a psychedelically repainted school bus, destination "FURTHUR," preaching a gospel of mental liberation through LSD, and blowing minds through California, across the sunbelt, and up to New York. There was a lot of marijuana around, too: Kesey would face possession charges and do jail time as a result. Tom Wolfe documented the whole thing, passionately engaging with the freaks without ever becoming one of them, and recording their adventures in vivid detail. If you want to know how Beatniks became hippies, and what being a hippie really meant—the radicalism, not just the long hair—then this is an essential read.

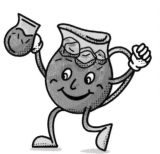

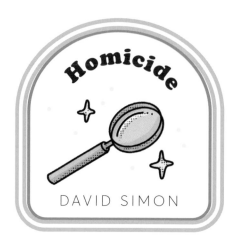

Homicide, by David Simon

One of the best true-crime books ever written, this is the pioneering account of the year a journalist spent shadowing homicide detectives in Baltimore. It's gripping, an eye-opening introduction to a city in the throes of a hard-drug epidemic—and the flawed, but often heroic, men (and they *are* nearly all men: the year was 1987) who were tasked with solving the murders that the drug trade caused. You'll never look at a cop show in the same way.

Killing Pablo, by Mark Bowden

A vivid account of the life and death of one of the world's most notorious drug dealers. Pablo Escobar ran the Medellín Cartel, defying the authorities for years and leaving a trail of bodies in his wake. Mark Bowden's account is full of surprising details: for instance, the police squad who finally shot Escobar dead immediately trimmed his prized mustache so that in photos taken of the body he would resemble Hitler.

Snowblind: A Brief Career in the Cocaine Trade, by Robert Sabbag

The true story of the career of pioneering cocaine dealer Zachary Swan, an ex-U.S. Marine who came up with a wide variety of scams to move drugs back in the days before the cartels took over, when you could do it with sharp wits and as little violence as possible. A globetrotting tale that was a bestseller on release and has long been accorded mythical status by literate drug dealers.

Loaded: A Misadventure on the Marijuana Trail, by Robert Sabbag

Sabbag followed up *Snowblind* with this account of the adventures of Allen Long, a marijuana smuggler who brought weed in from Colombia in the 1970s and 1980s. Again, it's packed with incidents and reads like a novel—making you nostalgic for a less-violent era of international drug trafficking.

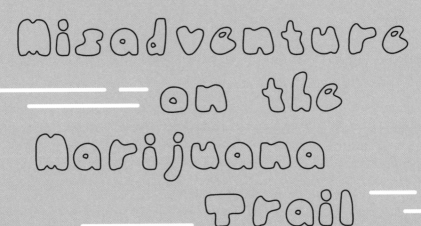

A Misadventure on the Marijuana Trail

Racing Reads

A bit of crime, a bit of peril, perhaps some violence... and, certainly, weed. These are reads to get the pulse racing. Enjoy them with a stimulating *sativa* smoke!

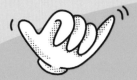

Fight Club, by Chuck Palahniuk

Don't worry if you've seen the movie; there's so much more to this than the big reveal—snapping dialogue, moments of chilling threat, and snippets of unusual information. Underneath it all lies an all-too-convincing argument that modern life's conveniences, niceties, and comforts are taking something fundamental away from us. While Palahniuk's characters may well be right about that, it's perhaps not the best idea to go bare-knuckle fighting in response; one is tempted to advise his anonymous protagonist to roll up a calming joint instead—as you should while you enjoy Palahniuk's rapid-fire prose, dark humor, and thought-provoking scenario.

The Taste of Metal, by Joe Hnida

Set in Denver's Capitol Hill neighborhood, this is a look at how one unconventional corner of society reacts to legalization of medical, and then recreational, marijuana. There's money to be made, but there are pitfalls, and Hnida's protagonist Jake doesn't miss them. With a dark undertone of bad love and seedy business, *The Taste of Metal* will show you a side of Denver that the tour operators probably won't.

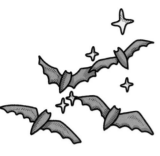

Fear and Loathing in Las Vegas, by Hunter S. Thompson

You've read this already, haven't you? If not, you probably should. Thompson found national fame in the late 1960s as one of the era's most distinctive writers, covering everything from sports to politics. *Fear and Loathing* is a novel, but it's based on two anarchic weekends Thompson spent in Las Vegas, ostensibly covering a motorcycle race but in practice dosing himself with every drug he could get his hands on, destroying hotel rooms, and speeding around the city. His aim was to get to the heart of the American dream and work out what had happened to the dreams and energies of the '60s counterculture: one can only conclude that he succeeded. The book has been a cultural reference point ever since, deservedly hailed as a classic, and is one of the most riotous reads of all time.

Trainspotting, by Irvine Welsh

Like Thompson, Welsh was a heavy drinker and drug user who lived the life he wrote about. Also like Thompson, his writing veers from horror to broad humor and back again, but he is, additionally, able to write in multiple voices and from different characters' points of view. Set in 1980s Edinburgh, *Trainspotting* tells the stories of a group of drug users who struggle with their families, their upbringing, unemployment, depression, addiction, and each other. Put like that, it sounds grim, but there is riotous humor throughout, and Welsh's inventive use of language and fearless engagement with the less-hygienic aspects of drug addiction made it a reference point for a generation, and a must-read today.

Inherent Vice, by Thomas Pynchon

Books with potheads as lead protagonists lend themselves to comedy. In this case, Larry "Doc" Sportello is a private eye, but not the regular kind: he's the kind who has to spray air-freshener in the office "on the off-chance his unknown visitor might take a dim view of his marijuana use." His case opens with a Chandleresque commission from a beautiful ex-girlfriend, asking him to protect her new lover from a devious plot—but, of course, it's not that simple. Sportello is soon spiraling through LA and Vegas, chasing down leads, running foul of the LAPD, and smoking a good deal of weed. Pynchon's most accessible, immediate book is a romp full of laughs and reveals, and is perfectly suited to a leisurely session in a hammock with a couple of reefers on hand.

Budding Prospects: A Pastoral, by T. Coraghessan Boyle

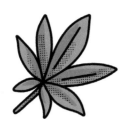

One rainy San Francisco night, directionless Felix Nasmyth receives a visit from an old buddy, Vogelsang, who has an offer: grow two thousand marijuana plants and get paid half a million dollars for it. Too good to be true, right? Of course it is, and in this early novel Boyle has a good deal of fun lining his entrepreneurial heroes up against a variety of enemies, ranging from the California Highway Patrol to a bear and the neighbors. It's a romp, undeservedly neglected, and will almost make you feel nostalgic for the bad old days of criminalization. Almost.

Go-Between, by Lisa Brackmann

A gripping thriller in which no one is who they say they are, set amid California's weed trade, dirty local politics, prison rackets, and a manipulative CIA agent. The dark side of the growth in growing…

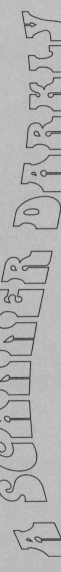

A *Scanner Darkly*, by Philip K. Dick

Although many of the characters smoke pot in this chilling vision of a future war on drugs, it isn't the drug that drives the plot of the book: that is Substance D, a powerful (imaginary, thankfully) psychoactive that splits the mind in two. Bob Arctor is using it, dealing it, and at the same time covertly informing on his fellow users to the police. The police aren't what they seem, either, and as Bob gradually loses it, the reader starts to see a sinister bigger picture. Dick had lived with heavy drug users for some time when he wrote this (and had himself been addicted to amphetamine), and there's an atmosphere of suspicion, paranoia, and mistrust that feels all too real throughout. One to convince you to stay on the pot…

King Suckerman, by George Pelecanos

Pelecanos writes about the fluid border between innocent hustles and small-time crime like no one else. Nearly all his books are brilliant and nearly all of them have a certain whiff of pot smoke. *King Suckerman*, perhaps, stands out from the rest, and hinges on a drug deal gone wrong.

Mid Ocean, by T. Rafael Cimino

An account of both sides of the 1980s war on drugs, this intricate story has been praised by a host of Miami veterans of the scene—ex-smugglers and ex-cops alike—who testify to its accuracy and the depth of Cimino's research. And you'll learn a lot about how to transport drugs by boat.

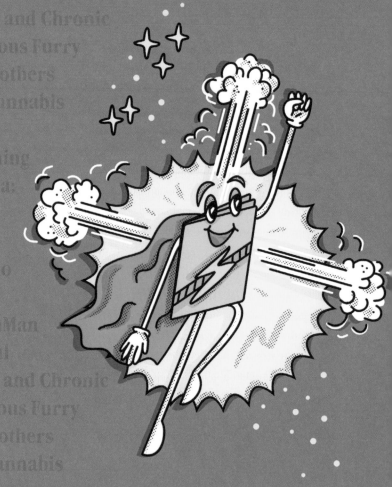

Comic Books

Comic books are by their nature somewhat less demanding on the brain than their purely verbal counterparts: the pictures give you something to enjoy even when your faculties are too compromised for the tricky art of reading actual words. So it's no surprise that, since weed went widespread back in the 1960s, a host of distinctive voices—ranging from the crude to the spiritual—have used the comic medium to make stories for lovers of the chronic. Over the years, too, the simple comic book has taken on an often-iconic status with the classification of the "graphic novel," lifting this medium that was once viewed as something for kids and sci-fi nerds to become its own art form. So whether you're looking for high art, kids' comedy, a politically provoking piece, or just something to while away the weedy hours, there's something for everyone, and every mood. If you need a bit of help to get you started on the huge array that's on offer, here are ten that stand out…

Comic books are by their nature somewhat less demanding on the brain than their purely verbal counterparts.

The pictures give you something to enjoy even when your faculties are too compromised for the tricky art of reading actual words.

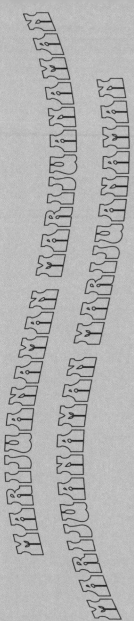

MarijuanaMan, by Ziggy Marley

You'd imagine that Bob Marley's son would not only know his way around a joint but also be a passionate advocate for weed's benefits. In this graphic novel—with distinctive art from Jim Mahfood—he introduces an extraterrestrial champion, MarijuanaMan, who promises to liberate the world not only from the evil clutches of PharmaCon's "synthetic pleasure chemicals" but also the supervillain Cash Money. One to enjoy if you're one of those stoners who sees the weed as a sacred route to global emancipation.

Mr. Natural, by Robert Crumb

One of the most enduring creations of the prolific, problematic comic artist Robert Crumb, Mr. Natural started giving us the benefit of his wisdom back in the 1960s. Satirizing the gurus of the day, the bearded sage meanders happily through life, offering such wisdom as "The secret of life is… hang loose!" to a changing cast of acolytes (including Crumb himself) but never quite achieving transcendental grace.

Bluntman and Chronic, by Kevin Smith

Spinning off from Kevin Smith's classic stoner movie *Clerks*, *Bluntman and Chronic* tells the story of Jay and Silent Bob's superhero alter-egos. They live in the Bluntcave, they drive a Bluntmobile, they fight with Bluntsabers… but, frankly, they aren't that great at the whole superhero thing. As perhaps you'd expect. Fortunately, their adversaries, the magnificently named League of Shitters, are pretty incompetent, too…

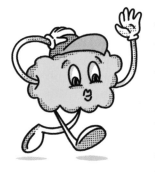

The Fabulous Furry Freak Brothers, by Gilbert Shelton

Created by a Texan college dropout in 1969, the Freak Brothers were not only a reflection of '60s counterculture, but also defined its hippie archetypes. Freewheelin' Franklin Freek was the cowboy-booted drifter; Phineas T. Phreak, the left-wing Beatnik intellectual; Fat Freddy Freekowtski, the slobbish, munchie-oriented incompetent. Together with Fat Freddy's Cat, they spent decades trying to score, trying not to get busted, traveling the world—and never quite getting around to cleaning their apartment. The stories are romps, with some antiestablishment satire, but none of the edge (or misanthropy) of Robert Crumb's contemporary work. They are all still in print today, giving you a heady whiff of '60s nostalgia suffused with the spirit of the stoner's classic adage: "Dope will get you through times of no money, better than money will get you through times of no dope."

Captain Cannabis, by Verne Andru

The passion project of Verne Andru, a Canadian animator who has worked with such "straight" giants as Disney and Hanna-Barbera, *Captain Cannabis* started life as a self-published monochrome Xerox. Forty years later, it's in color, and the scope of the titular hero's adventures has broadened. Once a lovelorn down-and-out roadie, now he's a superbeing, able—with the aid of the herb—to physically manifest his thoughts, but, unfortunately, he's also caught up in an extradimensional struggle for planet Earth. It is, in fact, a transcendent adventure: as Andru puts it, "He goes through a spiritual awakening by smoking pot… when you get into the higher realms of spiritualism there is a point where you have to ask 'what is the real truth?'" One for the astral travelers among us…

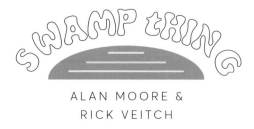

ALAN MOORE &
RICK VEITCH

Swamp Thing, by Alan Moore and Rick Veitch

Ostensibly a horror comic, but one that's packed with soul and a love of all things green, *Swamp Thing* made Alan Moore's name in the U.S., and his run on the DC strip remains a classic nearly forty years later. Abandoning the comic code regulations, the series dealt with all kinds of adult themes, but underpinning it all is a very weed-friendly preoccupation with the ecology and the spirit. There's plenty here: you can disappear into the swamp for a few days at a stretch, and come out again thoroughly changed…

Tank Girl, by Alan Martin and Jamie Hewlett

Emerging from the punky underground in the late 1980s, *Tank Girl* inspired a legion of young fans to shave their heads, smoke heavily, and drive tanks around the irradiated Australian outback. Well, two out of three ain't bad. She remains a uniquely *different* heroine: irreverent, anarchic, foul-mouthed, and violent, with a supporting cast including several talking stuffed toys and a mutant kangaroo boyfriend, the devoted Booga. The whole thing is bonkers, but the strips are packed with detail and humor, tightly plotted, and well worth an afternoon of your time and a little of your stash. (There was a movie, too, which you really don't need to see.)

Ex Machina: Smoke Smoke, by Brian K. Vaughan and Tony Harris

Set in a roughly speaking realistic version of New York, this episode of the long-running series takes a good look at the issue of decriminalization—from the point of view of those doing the decriminalizing. Ex-superhero Mitchell Hundred is now the city's mayor, who has to consider ups and downs of reforming the drug laws while dealing with a host of other issues. No one writes grown-up adventure comics like Vaughan, and this is some of his best work.

Little Nemo, by Winsor McCay

One of the most inventive comic strips was one of the very first. Published in the first decades of the twentieth century, McCay's charming one-page strips recount the gentle dream adventures of a young boy as he explores fantastical versions of the island of Manhattan. Smoke yourself into a reverie and slip into the gorgeous illustrations of Nemo's nocturnal visions.

From Hell, by Alan Moore and Eddie Campbell

One for the paranoid among us, one for the conspiracy theorist, one for the horror fan, this is a dark imagining of the events around the Jack the Ripper murders. In Alan Moore's reconstruction, which draws heavily on contemporary sources but is definitely fiction, the killer is instructed to carry out the murders in order to protect the highest levels of society from scandal. His true motivation, though, is more esoteric—even visionary. Gull's chilling amorality, and the darkness and poverty of Victorian London, are vividly captured in Eddie Campbell's scratchy, monochrome art; richly deserving of the many awards it won, *From Hell* is a perfect late-night, smoky read.

Amsterdam, the Netherlands
Brighton, U.K.
Catalonia, Spain
Ibiza, Spain
Lisbon, Portugal
Hamburg, Germany
Prague, Czech Republic
Kanepi, Estonia
Chefchaouen, Morocco
Vancouver, Canada
Montreal, Canada
Denver, Colorado
San Francisco,
 California
Portland, Oregon
Burlington,
 Vermont
Kingston, Jamaica
Cuzco, Peru
Montevideo, Uruguay
Phnom Penh, Cambodia
North Korea
Kathmandu, Nepal
Varanasi, India
Cape Town, South Africa
Gold Coast, Australia
Nimbin, Australia

Come fly with me!

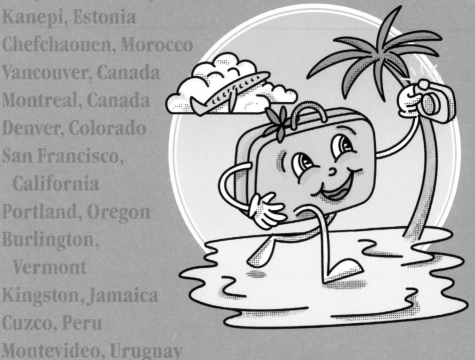

Travel

Travel broadens the mind, they say, and nothing will enrich your experience of a new spot better than a thoughtful smoke of the local weed.

Travel broadens the mind, they say, and nothing will enrich your experience of a new spot, nor ingratiate you with the *sativa*-smoking natives, better than a thoughtful toke of the local weed. The following is a selection of global destinations that have been chosen with smoking in mind—from established, relaxed dope destinations like Denver and Amsterdam, where you can be sure of an uninterrupted smoke, to some less obvious spots like Varanasi, India, and Nimbin, in Australia, who will turn a liberal blind eye to your buzz. Just make sure that you are up to date on the local legal situation before you start asking for sellers or lighting up in public. While the global trend is increasingly toward legalization or at least decriminalization, discretion and accountability are absolutely advised in all locations, or you might not be seeing much more of your destination than the inside of the local police cell.

Listed by continent, here is a selection of destinations that have been chosen with smoking in mind.

Amsterdam, the Netherlands

For decades the world capital of relaxed and legal marijuana use, the infamous Dutch city remains an amazing destination for global smokers.

Although the number of coffee shops legally selling marijuana is in fact in long-term decline all over the Netherlands, there are still more than 500 in the country, of which approximately 170 are in the nation's capital, Amsterdam—so you're spoiled for choice. They are subject to regulation, but nothing that will stop you from having a great time, and the sheer variety and quality of their offering, plus the many other fascinating cultural sights of the city, mean that you simply have to go at some point in your life.

The best way to enjoy the city is to plan to take in the streets, museums, galleries, and other sights in the morning (when your natural levels of cortisol are high, making you more alert and less receptive to cannabinoids), and to settle down to enjoy a smoke in the late afternoon. Rather than the tourist-trap joints in the red-light district, why not head to one of the less-central cafés, where you're more likely to meet friendly locals (and less likely to be kicked out when the proprietors want to clear your table): the Smoke Palace by the Oosterpark, Ruthless on the west side of town, or Katsu to the south.

Most cafés offer a wide range of different strains to smoke, with knowledgeable staff ("budtenders") able to direct you toward the best buzz, and of course there are plenty of cakes and bakes to try, and sweet drinks and treats to stave off the munchies. Remember when ordering that Dutch people are famously no-nonsense and direct— so don't take offence or mistake blunt statements of fact for rudeness—and also that it's illegal to combine marijuana with tobacco or alcohol.

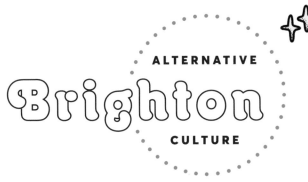

ALTERNATIVE

CULTURE

Brighton, U.K.

One of the capitals of alternative culture in the U.K., Brighton hasn't legalized or decriminalized weed, but the locals don't seem to have noticed, and it is common to see or smell them smoking it on the streets. Worth visiting for that, it's also known for its vibrant music scene, and the beachfront.

Catalonia, Spain

Since 2017, marijuana has been legal in this corner of Spain, with a thumping majority of legislators supporting legalization for members of cannabis clubs—which are limited to producing 330 pounds of weed each year. And Catalonia is a beautiful, fascinating part of the world. So what's the hitch? Well, they don't want you. Officials in Barcelona fear that an influx of toking tourists will turn the city into a seedy Amsterdam-style destination, so members have to wait two weeks after joining a cannabis club before they can actually buy some themselves. All the more reason to make friends with a local!

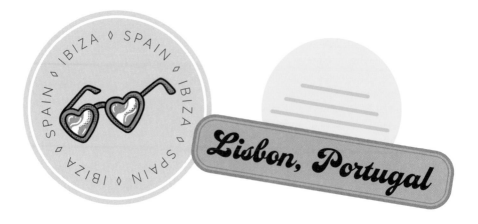

Ibiza, Spain

Europe's playground, Ibiza is a small island that plays host to millions upon millions of visitors every year and celebrates its unabashed attitude toward hedonism of all kinds. Avoid the hard-drinking tourist traps of San Antonio and explore the beautiful coastline and countryside instead for stimulating smokes in the open air.

Lisbon, Portugal

You won't get into trouble smoking weed here, so long as you're not provocative about it, but you may have to fight your way past some of the world's most mediocre "drug" dealers to find anything that's actually worth smoking. A thriving class of scammers approaches tourists, offering them nice bud on the street… too good to be true, right? Of course, these people are notorious for selling lumps of oregano or bay leaf as weed. Finding good weed or hash is trickier than you might think: make friends with someone in your hotel—not on the street, or online.

Hamburg, Germany

Germany is very relaxed about weed in general—it's decriminalized, and discreet use won't get you into trouble—and Hamburg is famously the most relaxed city in Germany. Score a little in one of the parks and enjoy it somewhere with a view of the ships coming and going to the container port. Then spend the evening enjoying the city's thriving music scene and bar-hopping.

Prague, Czech Republic

Another European city where the bud is tolerated if not officially encouraged, Prague has a liberal, welcoming feel and a hopping bar culture. Don't buy on the streets (unless you want oregano), but feel free to ask bar staff or friendly locals where you can score. When you succeed, enjoy walking around this beautiful city with your buzz on, taking in the sights before enjoying a local beer.

Kanepi, Estonia

Have some sympathy for this small town in a remote corner of Estonia—itself a small country tucked into a corner of the Baltic Sea. Like many places in Eastern Europe (Chernobyl is another), this place takes its name from a plant that grew freely there in earlier times. Kanepi means "hemp"—cannabis—and when the time came for the council to decide on a new coat of arms for the place, an online poll resoundingly voted for the familiar seven-pointed weed leaf. A degree of online trolling was suspected: 12,000 people voted, yet the local population is under half that. In any case, marijuana smoking, while not legal, is tolerated, and Estonia is a nice place to visit.

chefchaouen

Chefchaouen, Morocco

The Rif, a range of mountains in the northwestern corner of Africa, has long been one of the world's biggest producers of hashish—known locally as *kif*—and Chefchaouen is the regional center of the trade. It's also a famously beautiful city, with busy markets, interesting local products to buy, and plenty of places to stay. Beware, though: smoking is still illegal here, so be discreet about it—seek advice from the place where you stay.

Vancouver, Canada

While the whole nation is now pretty cannabis-friendly, Vancouver is definitely one of Canada's hottest spots for smokers. Head for an officially licensed dispensary, pick up some BC bud, then (if the weather's fine) head for Wreck Beach, on the edge of the city—North America's largest naturist location. Get high, be nude, enjoy the sun and the air on your skin!

Montreal, Canada

The magic letters? SQDC: *Société québécoise du cannabis*. These are the government-run stores where you can pick up your recreational weed. To smoke it, though, is another matter: there is a looooong list of forbidden zones, which includes anywhere within 30 feet of the entrance to any private or public building. That said, the locals are liberal, and in summertime you can easily find a spot with a riverside view and get your buzz on.

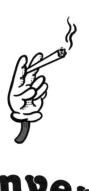

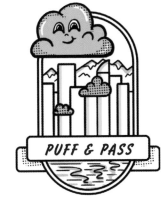

Denver

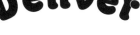

COLORADO
U.S.A.

Denver, Colorado

Check out the mile-high city for a glimpse of what late-period capitalism will look like when marijuana is allowed to play a full legal role in the economy.

The beauty of Colorado isn't just that there are numerous establishments where you can legally smoke, it's the good-natured support economy that has grown up around them. While regulations around business have shifted continually, making it difficult for cafés, clubs, restaurants, and so on to establish themselves, it is legal to smoke in a private home, and easy to buy at a dispensary. A host of other businesses have taken advantage of this, so when you visit, try out Puff, Pass, and Paint (a painting class with cannabis), Puff, Pass, and Pottery (a pottery class with cannabis), Bend and Blaze (a yoga class with cannabis), Colorado Cannabis tours (a tour bus with… you get the picture, right?), or any one of a huge number of other experiences. One day—probably not in the far future—every big city in the U.S. will be like this…

San Francisco, California

The home of many of the legalization movement's leading lights, from Brownie Mary onward, San Francisco is now home to a thriving legal smoke scene, with upmarket dispensaries springing up and catering to recreational and medical marijuana smokers alike.

Portland, Oregon

This is a vision of the future: what the world's cities will be like when marijuana is legalized everywhere. You can shop for it at upmarket dispensaries, you can stay in weed-friendly "bud-and-breakfast" accommodations, you can buy entire wardrobes of hemp couture, and you can find a wide variety of cannabis-oil moisturizers to boot.

Burlington, Vermont

Recreational cannabis is legal in Vermont, and the city is notable for the support it offers budding weed farmers: several specialist stores offer high levels of expertise which will help you get growing, rather than simply grinning on a couch.

Kingston, Jamaica

Ganja is, of course, an important part of Jamaican culture and the local Rastafarian religion. The government belatedly woke up to this in 2015, decriminalizing possession of small quantities. Since that time, some medical marijuana dispensaries have opened up, and some enterprising plantation owners offer tours of their crops. Be careful not to overdo it, though; the local landrace bud is strong, and it's easy to enjoy too much by accident.

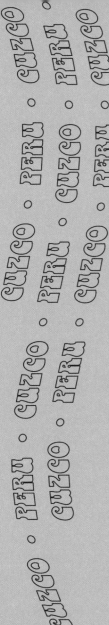

Cuzco, Peru

There's no long tradition of marijuana in Peru, but it has decriminalized possession of small amounts of the drug, and Cuzco is an excellent place to enjoy some. The combination of indigenous culture and Spanish colonialism has resulted in a city that is loaded with history and unique sights. Be careful, though, as Cuzco is more than two miles above sea level (twice as high as Denver), and the air makes altitude sickness a common condition. Wait until you're acclimatized before you light up!

Montevideo, Uruguay

This small South American nation was a pioneer in legalizing marijuana, and if you're over eighteen you can smoke pot legally anywhere other than in a public building or enclosed place of work. At home, citizens can grow their own personal stash of up to six flowering female plants, or if they're feeling community-spirited, join a "Club de Cannabis," licensed to grow up to ninety-nine. The whole system is regulated by the post office—not the police— and results in high-quality pot costing approximately one-tenth of what it does in the U.S.

Phnom Penh, Cambodia

Not legalized, but laws against pot are barely enforced and as long as you don't smoke ostentatiously in public, you'll be fine. This contrasts with neighboring Thailand and Vietnam, where laws *are* enforced, making this the weed capital of Southeast Asia. Many places advertise "happy pizza"—which has grass liberally sprinkled over the cheese, and does the job nicely. The local weed is low quality but so cheap that it doesn't really matter. Plan to visit in mid-April, when the Khmer New Year is celebrated.

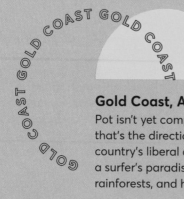

GOLD COAST GOLD COAST GOLD COAST GOLD COAST GOLD COAST

Gold Coast, Australia

Pot isn't yet completely decriminalized in Australia but that's the direction of travel. Make the most of the country's liberal attitudes by heading to Gold Coast, a surfer's paradise on the east coast, where long beaches, rainforests, and hundreds of miles of canals meet.

North Korea

It's a surprising fact that one of the most repressive societies in the world is entirely relaxed about cannabis. It grows wild everywhere, and many citizens cultivate a plant or two for their own use at home, using the low-strength harvest to wind down after another difficult day in one of the world's last communist dictatorships. That said, any kind of interaction with foreigners is discouraged, so you're unlikely to have a nice mellow bonding session with the locals.

Kathmandu, Nepal

Historically, Nepal was one of the centers of global weed production and distribution, with hippies flocking to its capital, Kathmandu, to enjoy safe, legal, local highs. That ended in 1973 when Nixon told the government to criminalize cannabis, a strategy that backfired badly as heroin traffickers moved in. These days it's easy to buy weed or hash, but it's a sleazy street-corner business. There is, though, a viable ethical-hemp industry here, and much else to enjoy in this beautiful country: trekking, culture, and food—so it is well worth a visit.

VARANASI

Varanasi, India

The city is sacred to Hindus, Buddhists, and Jains alike, and like many places in India's northern provinces, has a comfortable relationship with cannabis—known as *bhang*. Possibly the best way to enjoy it is to have a *bhang lassi* from one of the many licensed stores that sell it, and sit yourself on one of the spectacular *ghats*—stepped embankments that line the holy River Ganges. Your buzz may last several hours, and the constant boat traffic will become more fascinating as it progresses...

Cape Town, South Africa

Regularly voted one of the best places in the world to visit, Cape Town has a relaxed attitude toward smoking and is surrounded by amazing spots with spectacular views. The coastline has beaches, caves, and penguin colonies, and famed Caribbean restaurant Trenchtown has regular 420-themed nights.

Nimbin, Australia

This tiny cattle town in a remote corner of New South Wales has, since 1973, pretty much been run by the freaks. Working in partnership with the local indigenous communities, they have hosted festivals, made great strides toward sustainable living, and, in effect, informally legalized cannabis—of which they grow huge quantities locally.

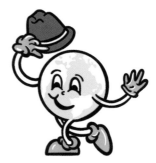

High Times Cannabis Cup
The Emerald Cup
National Cannabis Festival
Nimbin MardiGrass
Cannabis Expo
  and Convention
Hash Bash
Pan Ram
420 Hyde Park
Seattle Hempfest
Electric Highway
SPLIFF Film
  Festival
Glastonbury
  Festival
Hanfparade
  Berlin
Stepping High Festival
420 Hippie Hill
420 Toronto
FlyHi 420 Denver
420 Vancouver
Roskilde
Great Midwest Marijuana Harvest Festival
Austin Reggae Festival
Burning Man
Las Vegas Hemp Festival

Events

At these dedicated events, you might meet like-minded smokers, learn about the latest developments in breeding and growing, and be a visible part of promarijuana activism.

It can be lonely smoking on your own, or even with the same old faces. Why not get off the couch and head for one of the annual smoke-ins? At these dedicated events, you might meet like-minded smokers, learn about the latest developments in breeding and growing, and be a visible part of promarijuana activism. It is also an opportunity to lend your voice to campaigns for freedom, and to protest against the unjust incarceration of too many people who are still doing time for enjoying cannabis. Whichever you head for, you can party, too! Some of these events are explicitly dope-friendly; at others, some discretion would be sensible.

Why not get off the couch and head for one of these annual smoke-ins?

High Times Cannabis Cup

Undoubtedly the highest-profile event in the field, this has grown from being a modest affair in Amsterdam to a huge carnival that draws massive crowds across the States. (Varying locations.)

The Emerald Cup

Drawing huge crowds from across the nation, this three-day California festival covers everything: the business, the music, the medicine, the horticulture… and a beer garden. To which the police have not been called once in thirteen years of the event. (Sonoma, CA, December.)

National Cannabis Festival

The motto: celebrate; educate; activate. This one-day festival features top-drawer live music and plenty of advocacy, education, and activism aimed at reforming the law in and around Washington, D.C. (Washington, D.C., April.)

Nimbin MardiGrass

This Australian festival has its roots in an egg-based protest against undercover police operations. Every year since 1993, this festival has celebrated the weed in all its forms, and is notable for the Growers Ironperson event, in which—in tribute to the many local weed farmers—the contestants must first run with a 44lb sack of fertilizer, then a bucket of water, and then a marijuana plant. (Nimbin, N.S.W., Australia, May.)

The Cannabis Expo

A business-oriented expo accompanies a political and economic convention. Probably less fun than many other of the listed events, but playing its part in the development of the cannabis business nonetheless. (Cape Town, South Africa, October.)

Hash Bash

A civil protest with a long history, the Ann Arbor Hash Bash is an hour-long protest held each year at the University of Michigan. Speeches, music, activism, occasional civil disobedience. (Ann Arbor, MI, April.)

Pan Ram

The participants in the Hash Bash have achieved many of their aims: the founders of this Thai marijuana festival, which started in 2019, have that same long road ahead of them as they aim to change attitudes, build the local marijuana economy, and release the health benefits. (Pan Ram Thailand, usually takes place in April.)

420 Hyde Park

One of many, many informal smoke-ins that take place each April 20, this is the U.K.'s largest. Thousands attend, but there's not much for them to do except enjoy the spring sunshine, relax in the Royal Park, and skin up. And that's just fine. (London, U.K., April—obviously.)

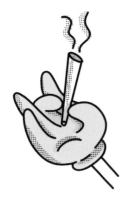

Seattle Hempfest

Probably the largest festival of its kind in the world, Hempfest regularly draws 100,000 people over three days. Legalization hasn't taken the wind out of its sails: crowds get larger every year, and it now has five stages spread along Seattle's waterfront. (Seattle, WA, August.)

Electric Highway

Evolving out of a regular 420 festival, Calgary's Electric Highway promises "two days of killer bands, rad artists, and fuzzy vibes." Expect alt-rock, beer, and plenty of weed. (Calgary, Canada, April.)

SPLIFF Film Festival

Promising films that explore the meaning, pleasures, and culture of recreational marijuana use, this hasn't been going long but already has a keen following—and as every movie has to be less than four minutes and twenty seconds long, nothing will test your attention span. (Tours the West Coast in April–May, and online.)

Glastonbury Festival

Not, strictly speaking, a marijuana festival, but there is a huge range of hemp-and-cannabis-themed stalls and events. This is where the U.K. counterculture plays every year—all 210,000 of them. (Glastonbury, U.K., June.)

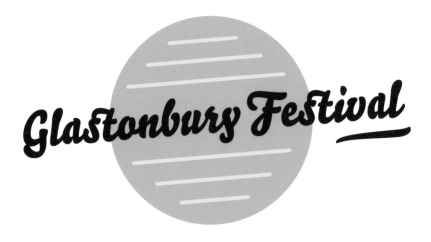

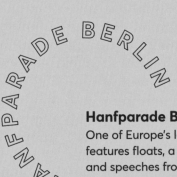

Hanfparade Berlin

One of Europe's largest legalization events, this features floats, a march through the center of the city, and speeches from a variety of experts. Police do not trouble those who smoke openly at the march. (Berlin, Germany, August.)

Stepping High Festival

Jamaica's leading ganja event, this aims to educate and entertain in equal measure. A competition assesses Jamaica's best farmer and best strain, attendees get plenty of opportunity to sample the entries, and there are forums, panel discussions, and a *lot* of reggae. (Negril, Jamaica, March.)

420 Hippie Hill

Billed as the first and biggest of the many 420 events that occur each year, this free festival occupies a sizable chunk of Golden Gate Park and fills the air above it with a palpable cloud of aromatic smoke. No kids, no booze— plenty of food if you get the munchies, though... (San Francisco, CA, April.)

420 Toronto

For many years this was a protest in front of City Hall. These days, with pot no longer a criminal matter, it has become more of a celebration and takes place on the shores of Lake Ontario. The whole city gets into the spirit; there are accompanying comedy, film, and music festivals at the same time. (Toronto, Canada, April.)

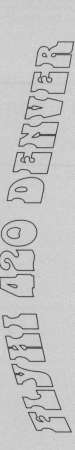

FlyHi 420 Denver

Already one mile high, and then they gather one of the largest crowds of smokers in the world… Denver's weed scene is transforming the city and this is one of the biggest, and smokiest of all the 420 fests. (Denver, CO, April.)

Great Midwest Marijuana Harvest Festival

This sounds like it should be bucolic and rural, but in fact it's a long-running street protest that aims to educate, inform, and reform the law under the serious headline: "Cannabis Prohibition Kills." There are bands and music, but it's less of a party than some other events. (Madison, WI, October.)

420 Vancouver

For more than twenty years, Vancouver's 420 has been celebrating cannabis culture. Attendance exceeds 150,000, and the event is notable for its farmers' market, showcasing the finest in local production. (Vancouver, Canada, April.)

Roskilde

One of the largest of the European music festivals, Roskilde has a laid-back, anarchic vibe and incredible acts. It has much in common with Glastonbury: set over several days, huge numbers of people, huge amounts of mud, huge amounts of weed. Enjoy! (Roskilde, Denmark, June–July.)

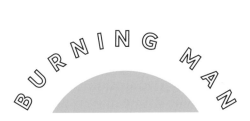

like-minded creative souls

Austin Reggae Festival

Unity in the community! Reggae, dancehall, Afrobeat, and more—the perfect accompaniment to a happy weekend of smoking. This annual event benefits the Central Texas Food Bank. No camping, unfortunately, so you have to be together enough to leave the grounds each evening. (Austin, TX, April.)

Burning Man

Craziness in the desert. This is where America gets its weird out. Lots of fire, lots of unusual scenes, plenty of music, plenty of art, plenty of opportunities to get properly high and collaborate (participation is key) with some like-minded creative souls. (Black Rock City, NV, September.)

Global Marijuana March

On the first weekend in May, smokers take to the streets all around the world. Marches have taken place simultaneously in cities as far apart as Copenhagen, Toronto, Paris, Vancouver, New York... There will likely be one near you; seek it out and join in!

The welcome home wind-down
Doing the do (after doing a doobie)
Doing a doobie (after doing the do)
Countryside hike'n'smoke
Pair meditations
Bathtime
Q and A
Marijuana
 massage
Musical
 mystery tour
Stoned shooting-
 star-gazing
The welcome
 home wind-down
Doing the do (after
 doing a doobie)
Doing a doobie (after doing the do)
Countryside hike'n'smoke

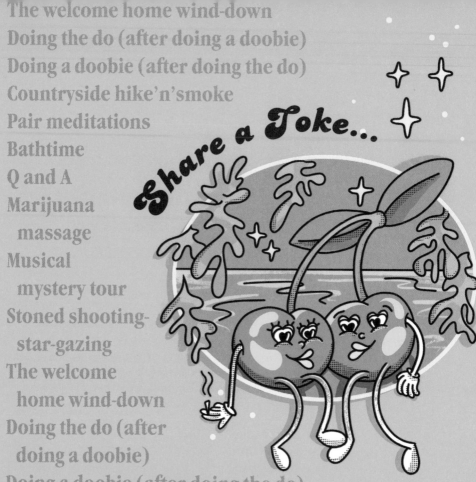

Share a Toke...

Relationships & Intimacy

Bathtime
Q and A
Pair meditations
Marijuana massage
Musical mystery tour

Recent research finds that for men and women alike, marijuana use increases the number of "intimacy events."

Smoking with your lover is... *smoking.*

Smoking alone is good; smoking with friends is better; smoking with your lover is… well, *smoking*. Knowing this, ever more couples have now discovered the benefits of enjoying cannabis together, in part as the perfect way to wind down from the stresses and strains of our hectic lifestyles and reconnect as a couple. In fact, recent research from the University at Buffalo finds that for men and women alike, marijuana use increases the number of "intimacy events" that they engage in—which can be any demonstration of love, caring, or support. Sharing a toke can also be an excellent way to prepare yourselves to discuss, debate, or offload any of those tricky issues that are bothering you, or that you've been putting off, calmly and without negativity or aggression. The right *sativa* strain will lower boundaries, reduce inhibitions, and allow us to rediscover a sense of joy and contentment. From simple evenings spending quality time together chilling, to activities to get you talking and sharing, here are a few ideas for creating an intimate oasis of affection and relaxation. And, if you like, a few more ideas to set the scene for an erotic oasis of profound sensuality…

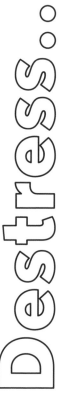

Destress...

The welcome home wind-down

Life, with its competing demands, is hard, and external pressures—be they professional, medical, family, social, or financial—can put great stresses on us and the people we love. It can be really difficult to leave those external pressures at the front door and greet our partner with positivity every day—and this negativity can swiftly become problematic, by making us difficult to live with. If that is the case, you can address it easily; as soon as you are both home in the evening, make a comfortable spot, and have a mild smoke dedicated to nothing but winding down, sidelining whatever's troubling you, and enjoying being with each other. Cannabinoids will reduce aggression and stress, letting you talk about difficult subjects without losing control or arguing. That's not to say that you shouldn't discuss whatever's on your mind, of course, but this way you can do it when you're relaxed, and not let the conversation be dominated by negative emotions.

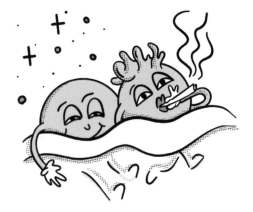

DOING THE DO...
DOING A DOOBIE

Doing the do (after doing a doobie)

Sex is, of course, a crucial component to most relationships, and weed's sensual and bonding properties make it a natural catalyst for the kind of rich, emotional lovemaking that will have you both feeling freshly reconnected and smiling for days. Make sure that you have the time to really get into the experience—tell each other how much you are anticipating it, then head for the bedroom, spark up, hold each other tight, and let nature take its course! You may find that your bodies are more attuned to the physical sensations of intimacy, that you're more emotional, and that you're less inhibited and more communicative. It's all good! And, even better, academic research has found that cannabinoids are equal-opportunity aphrodisiacs, increasing both male and female libido.

Doing a doobie (after doing the do)

If you've not indulged beforehand, a smoke after sex is an excellent way to maintain the precious intimacy that you've created. Post orgasm, your bodies will be swimming with dopamine, oxytocin, prolactin, vasopressin, and serotonin—all of the brain's own good-time chemicals, basically—which perfectly complement the cannabinoids of a smoke, prolonging and intensifying those feelings of shared love, connection, and satisfaction.

Countryside hike'n'smoke

Combining a healthy, refreshing countryside walk with a relaxing joint is an excellent way to make the most of both. Walk a few miles, climb a hill so that there's a view to enjoy, spread out the picnic blanket, and spark up a doobie. Pay attention to the sound of the birdsong, the wind in the trees, and the sensations of gentle exercise. Just be careful not to start any fires—and remember to take your trash home with you!

Bathtime

It's fun to slip into the tub with your loved one, and a mild high will turn it into a real treat. Wet fingers will quickly make a joint unpalatable, so you might want to take the brownie route and really luxuriate in the sensation of water on skin…

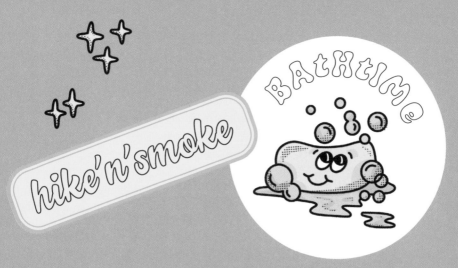

QUESTIONS & ANSWERS

Q and A

Remember those long, intense conversations that you had back when you first met? When you were getting to know each other and were fascinated to discover one another's personal philosophies, beliefs, loves, hates, turn-ons and turn-offs? When was the last time you had a conversation like that? If it was yesterday, congratulations. If you haven't had a really deep and meaningful conversation for a while, though, why don't you prepare some open-ended questions to ask each other while you're high and loquacious? Some examples to get you going: what is the accomplishment of which you are most proud? What age do you want to live to? Which dead person would you most like to meet? What are your three rules for life? What question do you most want to know the answer to? Who would you invite to your dream dinner party? Which fictional character do you feel closest to? It's best to prepare a long list before you start, but don't be surprised if just one of them takes you on a long conversation of shared discovery and insight.

Pair meditations

It can be fantastic to share a mindfulness meditation: you find yourself going on a journey with your loved one, and arriving together at a calm, intimate place. Why not try the marijuana meditation on pages 128–131? They will work just as well for a couple as a solo smoker.

Marijuana massage

A massage with CBD-infused oil won't get you high like a joint will, but it will be extremely good for the recipient and your relationship. CBD is a potent anti-inflammatory, and working it into the muscles and joints can bring deep pain relief and boosts of energy—as well as relaxation. The physical contact with a loved one is another benefit (you'll be flooding your body with love hormones like oxytocin), and those hormones in turn reduce stress and anxiety. Start with the shoulders and back, remembering to work each side symmetrically, then carry on to the legs, arms, and hands. Finish with the neck and scalp.

Stoned shooting-star-gazing

On a clear night, find the darkest, most remote spot you can. Set up a pair of beach recliners, cover yourself with a blanket if you need to, and sip a Thermos of hot chocolate while you smoke and watch the moon and stars above you. For your own shooting star show (sooo romantic!), use a meteor shower calendar to pick a night when there is likely to be more extraterrestrial activity. (Courtesy of the Draconids, Orionids, Leonids, and so on; there are meteor showers most months of the year.)

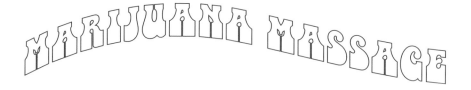

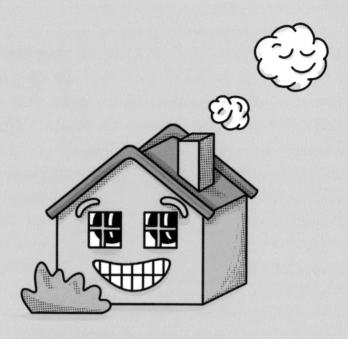

Musical mystery tour

This one takes a little preparation. Set aside an hour
together, no phones, in a darkened room with a good
stereo. One of you prepares an hour-long playlist of
carefully chosen tunes—music that will create a mood
and enhance the high. Choose songs that have stories
attached to them, songs that are particularly meaningful,
that have amazing musicianship or lyrics, or are exciting
new discoveries. Then just relax and listen through, talking
about the tunes as they come and go, but paying close
attention to them, appreciating each other's tastes, and
seeing where the journey takes you. The next time, it's the
other's turn to prepare the playlist.

Marijuana.com
Hightimes.com
MPP.org
Norml.org
Leafly.com
Howtogrowmarijuana.com
International Cannagraphic
   Magazine (icmag.com)
Rollitup.org
Marijuanadoctors.com
Weedmaps.com
Marijuanastocks.com
Kimmy Tan
Koala Puffs
MacDizzle
TheCCC420
That High Couple
Marijuana.com
Hightimes.com
Rollitup.org
MPP.org
Norml.org

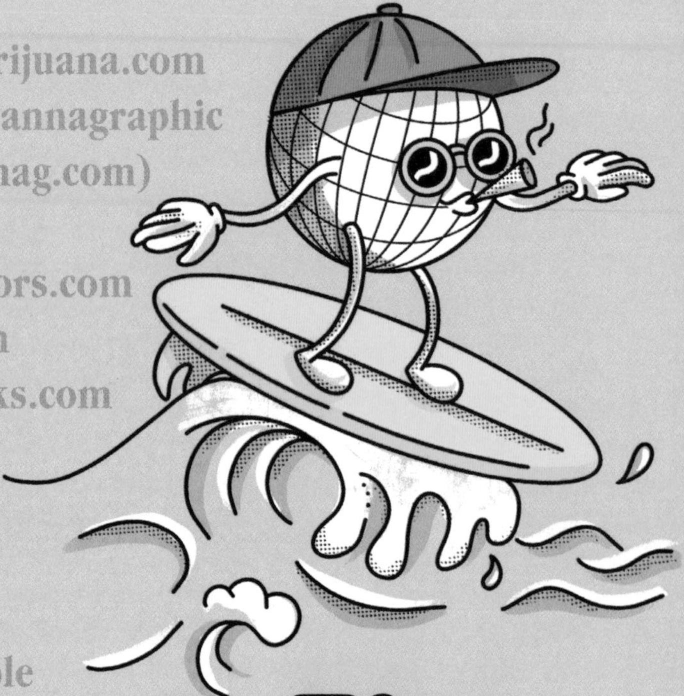

Leafly.com
Howtogrowmarijuana.com
Marijuanadoctors.com

The World Weed Web

An ashtray, a mouse, a keyboard, a screen… and where did the last four hours go, exactly? The web is full of rabbit holes that you can vanish into on any topic under the sun when you've got your smoke on (or even when you haven't, let's be honest!). But let's stay focused here. There are many, many weed-oriented websites out there on the *indica*net, and some are, as you can imagine, more interesting than others. Whether you want to know about the history of marijuana, the current views and rules about cannabis

The web is full of rabbit holes to vanish into when you've got your smoke on.

consumption, where to go for the best weed, what *is* the best weed, or if you want the amusement of watching other people get stoned on YouTube, it's all out there. If you can actually switch off the computer, you could even do something useful with all that surfing on the world weed web and learn how to cultivate your own cannabis crop. For those of you pushed for time (really?!), I've compiled the pick of the bunch; a selection of sites that are guaranteed to inform, entertain, educate, or appal—in a good way.

There are many, many weed-oriented websites out there on the indicanet, and some are more interesting than others.

Weedmaps.com

The *New York Times* of the weed scene, weedmaps.com is the place to go for in-depth law reporting, politics from a marijuana point of view, and lifestyle articles written by people who care about punctuation.

Hightimes.com

The voice of pot's radical past and progressive present, offering a similar balance of news and views to weedmaps.com, cultivation expertise, and sponsoring the Cannabis Cups as they proliferate across the U.S.A.

MPP.org

Dedicated to reform of the laws around marijuana, the Marijuana Policy Project is a serious campaigning body with the aim of changing law by supporting and co-ordinating efforts to influence policy and law enforcement.

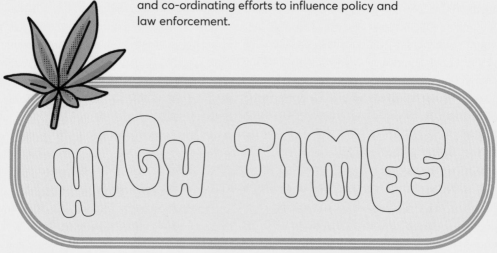

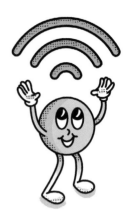

Norml.org

Website of the pioneering campaign organization, with similar resources to MPP.org and also encouraging you to take action or write directly to your representatives.

Leafly.com

An early example of the "professionalization" of the legal marijuana scene, Leafly presents thousands upon thousands of user reviews of strains and dispensaries, helping you find your way around the bewildering profusion of new buds, new stores, and new research.

Howtogrowmarijuana.com

A good one-stop shop for advice on growing indoors and out. It's been running since 1996 and the forums are a great source of support, comradeship, and expertise.

International Cannagraphic Magazine (icmag.com)

Another huge collection of forums and expertise. If your question's not already been answered here, then you're asking the wrong question…

Rollitup.org

Yet another collection of friendly forums to complete your knowledge base.

Marijuanadoctors.com and weedmaps.com

Similar gazetteers of all of the M.D.s currently working in this field, and of dispensaries nationwide.

Marijuanastocks.com

If you've got a few spare dollars and are looking for a weed-based investment, then come here: it offers stock picks, breaking news, and sector data.

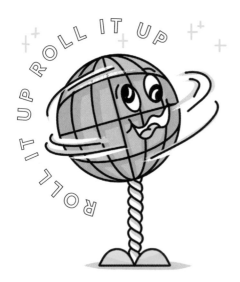

Californian Cannabis YouTube

Not so much a website as a colossal stoner-friendly rabbit hole, YouTube even decides what you want to watch next so you don't have to make even *that* basic decision yourself! Here are five stoner channels, based in legalized California, that are pretty much guaranteed to waste your time amusingly.

Kimmy Tan

Watch a heavily tattooed Los Angelena and her friends get stoned. She will try to sell you merchandise at the same time.

Koala Puffs

Watch a less-heavily tattooed Los Angelena and her friends get stoned. She occasionally involves her mother, and she will try to sell you merchandise, too.

MacDizzle

Watch a mid-level-tattooed Los Angelena and her friends, including Kimmy Tan and Koala Puffs, get stoned. Merchandise is available, obviously.

TheCCC420

The "Cannabis Connoisseur Connection" is more informative, less tattooed, and offers an interesting look inside California's marijuana industry. Strain reviews, etiquette guides, and less-manic video editing.

That High Couple

Neatly groomed, untattooed, and incredibly respectable-looking, Alice and Clark are married and consumer test all kinds of marijuana goods and goodies, reviewing equipment, stores, edibles, and more.

El Greco
Vincent van Gogh
Pablo Picasso
Georgia O'Keeffe
Mark Rothko
Salvador Dalí
Bridget Riley
Jackson Pollock
Hieronymus Bosch
Pieter Bruegel
 the Elder 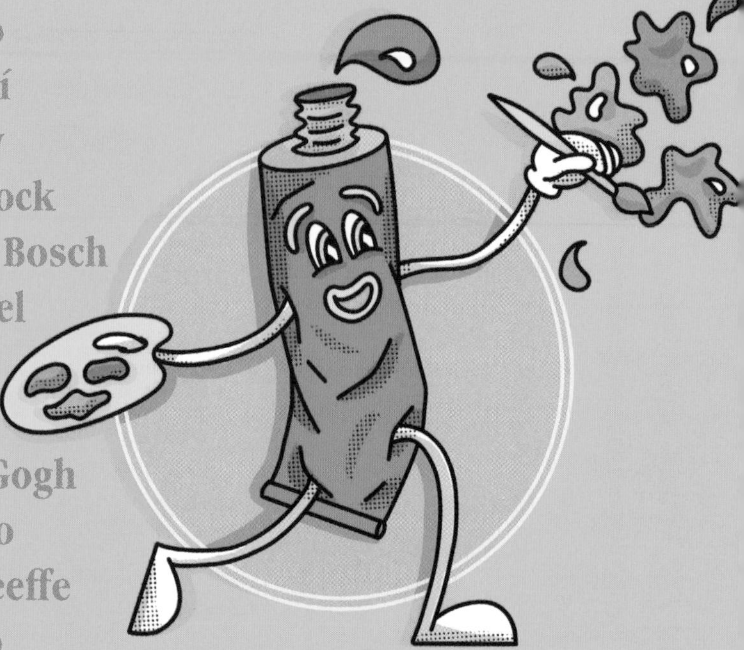
El Greco
Vincent van Gogh
Pablo Picasso
Georgia O'Keeffe
Mark Rothko
Salvador Dalí
Bridget
 Riley
Jackson
 Pollock
Hieronymus
 Bosch
Pieter Bruegel
 the Elder
El Greco
Vincent van Gogh

A Stoner's History of Fine Art

As Allen Ginsberg inspiringly noted in the lines that open this book, weed makes us more receptive to all kinds of stimulus, including sound, touch, and emotion. However, it's up to us to use this receptiveness creatively, giving our minds and souls the richest inputs that we can while we are in this altered state. Art-lovers will find a chilled smoke enables them to see things they've never seen before in a piece of art—the rest of us just might find that some of the more obscure canvases start to mean something, and they at last "get it." Whatever your preference—realism, naturalism, or the more abstract expressionist, surrealist, or just plain "out-there" art—light up, sit back, and allow yourself to be drawn into the images, to feel and see things differently, and to be inspired by another view. To this end, we have selected ten painters whose work will not only delight your eyes, but also feed your mind, broaden your artistic horizons, and present a history of stoner-friendly Western art. "Awe and detail," indeed.

Weed makes us more receptive to all kinds of stimulus: sound, touch, and emotion.

Art-lovers will find a chilled smoke enables them to see things they've never seen before in a piece of art.

Hieronymus Bosch

(c.1450–1516)

Only a few paintings by this Dutch master survive. He was born around 1450 in the south of Holland, but we know very little about him, except that he had one of the craziest, most balls-out imaginations of any painter: his best work is filled with creatures and deformed human figures that defy logic. Seek out *The Garden of Earthly Delights*, centered on a landscape whose buildings appear to be made from quivering pink flesh. Hundreds of naked sinners shamelessly display their bodies, or hide in giant eyeballs, ride overgrown songbirds, burst from eggs, gorge on gigantic fish and fruit, whip each other's backsides with flowers, and in general indulge every lustful impulse you can imagine, and a few that you probably can't. The same work's depictions of hell are, if anything, even more disturbing. Download the hi-res image, get yourself nice and mellow, and explore the garden at your leisure.

El Greco

(1541–1614)

Taking the conventions of Renaissance art and warping them in a distinctly expressionist direction, El Greco abandoned conventional measure and proportion in favor of movement and emotion. His human figures had distended features, exaggerated poses, and massive draped robes; his landscapes had dramatic, unnatural lighting and seem to sway as though in the grip of a gale. His paintings are the work of a man who was very happy to lose control. Look at *The Opening of the Fifth Seal*, with its warped figures ecstatically greeting the second coming, shedding their earthly robes and receiving the white robes of immortal saints; or *Laocoön*, showing the agonies of death by snakebite in a warped, dream-like world.

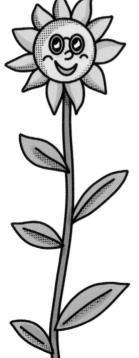

Vincent van Gogh

(1853–1890)

Many of van Gogh's key works find themselves in Amsterdam, a city that you probably want to visit anyway. When you've got yourself nicely buzzing, maybe on some edibles, take a look: the colors and compositions will blow you away. Van Gogh worked hard to understand color, which he endowed with profound emotional and spiritual qualities (yellow, for instance, stood for truth), and he painted it onto the canvas in thick smears and strokes that pull your eye along the line. He boldly applied contrasting dots and strokes of complementary colors that make the painting leap off the canvas, and are a feast for the eyes. Avoid his famous, and bilious, *Sunflowers*; instead, make for the landscapes—hot, luminous, inviting, vibrant.

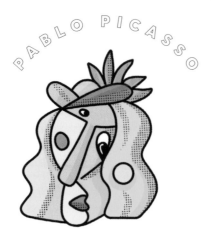

PABLO PICASSO

Pablo Picasso

(1881–1973)

Picasso worked in so many styles that he defies categorization. He left behind thousands of pieces of work, but all are agreed that there is one painting in particular that so abruptly broke with all the traditions of what had gone before that it marks a turning point in the history of art. Look at *Les Demoiselles d'Avignon*, a group painting of five nude prostitutes whose bodies are reimagined as flat, angular shapes, whose faces are distorted into masks, and whose emotionless eyes challenge the viewer unsettlingly. Picasso was obsessed by El Greco, but where his precursor had stretched and warped his human figures, Picasso seemed to cut them up and reassemble them. Painting multiple viewpoints onto one canvas, he would soon develop cubism—and revolutionize modern art. Be inspired by him to look at what you see differently, from several angles at once, to find beauty in ugliness—and ugliness in beauty.

Georgia O'Keeffe

Georgia O'Keeffe

(1887–1986)

A near-contemporary of Picasso, O'Keeffe was similarly obsessed with line, color, and form and had a long, successful career. She mastered conventional figurative painting before working for some years in abstracted forms, and created a highly distinctive oeuvre, which ranged from urban skyscapes to surreal juxtapositions of bones floating over desert landscapes. Look at *New York Street with Moon* to see sky and building cutting into each other, or *From the Faraway, Nearby* to understand her preoccupation with the arid New Mexico landscape. Her most famous works are her flower paintings, which celebrate curves, contours, and colors—and which are often seen in a profoundly sexual light. She never painted people, but her paintings are still full of humanity and life.

Mark Rothko

(1903–1970)

Bosch gives your roving eye thousands of places to land on each painting: there are details, people, movements, lines, textures. Rothko is the opposite. His paintings lack detail and are composed of floating rectangles and fields of color; they seem to move under our eyes, pulsing inward or outward. Rothko achieved these unique effects by thinly layering contrasting colors on top of one another; you can, for instance, look through a layer of red to see a layer of blue beneath. This gave his compositions an incredible vibrancy, and he added to that by scrubbing at the edges of his shapes with solvent, softening their edges and making them float in space. He wanted his paintings to inspire strong emotions, even tears. Get as close as you can to his canvases and allow yourself to be drawn in.

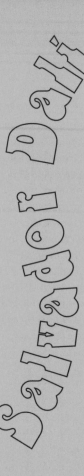

Salvador Dalí

(1904–1989)

Dalí was a surrealist, which meant that he was interested in accessing the subconscious brain—the part that throws up disturbing images in dreams—so his work definitely makes sense when you're high. He is the artist who first melted a clock, who married a lobster with a telephone, who used ants to express his profound sexual anxiety… and so on. Like Bosch, he filled his work with animals, lust, and impossible scenes, and like Bosch he was also profoundly (if unconventionally) religious. Find a trippy strain, don't be afraid to overdo it, and—like Dalí—try to push at your inhibitions as you appreciate his work.

Pieter Bruegel the Elder

(c.1525–1569)

If Bosch was interested in the fantastical, Bruegel (who was father and grandfather to a dynasty of artists bearing the same name) was preoccupied by the world around him. Thanks to his work, which has a *Where's Waldo?* level of activity and population, we have a vivid idea of what life in Renaissance Holland was actually like. We look down on towns and villages filled with activity: people fight, play, eat, drink, flirt, work, or just idle around the place. *The Peasant Wedding* fills a room with characters, stuffing themselves on food and beer; *Children's Games* populates a riotous town with anarchic kids; then, in an abrupt change of mood, *The Triumph of Death* takes a darker turn, showing an army of skeletons slaughtering their way across a blitzed landscape. Less hallucinatory than Bosch's work, but every bit as rewarding to pore over and explore.

Bridget Riley

(1931–present)

Riley's paintings don't show people, or landscapes, yet they burst with life all the same. The enormous "op-art" canvases that she produces use rhythmic patterns of carefully composed shapes and colors to play sophisticated tricks on your brain. Refusing to stay still as you look at them, her paintings shimmer, undulate, rotate, squeeze, and expand… Seek out the originals, if you can (or better, buy one for yourself: but you'll need a few million dollars to do so), get yourself good and high, and let your eyes vibrate on Riley's incredible wavelengths.

Jackson Pollock

(1912–1956)

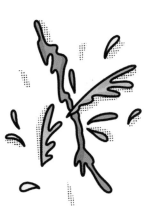

Another painter whose canvases are abstract assemblies of color, paint, and pattern, Pollock worked in a completely different way to Riley. Taking his huge canvases off the easel, he laid them on the floor and dripped and poured house paint over them, painting less with his eye than with his whole body, and recording gesture and motion. His paintings are not about the end result, but the artist's creative process; it's not about representing the external world, but his inner one. Look closely at the interactions of texture and color, and at the energy that the patterns of spills, drips, handprints, and splashes betray. Let yourself get sucked in, and picture the artist at work, stepping around the canvas and onto it, letting the chance fall of drops of paint speak for him.

Gratitude
Notice your breath
Tune in to your surroundings
Tune in to your body
Appreciate what
  you have
Fire and smoke
Inhalations
Feel the effects
Chants and
  mantras
Hugs and
  embraces
Notice your breath
Tune in to your surroundings
Tune in to your body
Appreciate what you have
Fire and smoke
Inhalations
Feel the effects
Chants and mantras
Hugs and embraces
Gratitude
Notice your breath
Tune in to your surroundings
Tune in to your body
Appreciate what you have

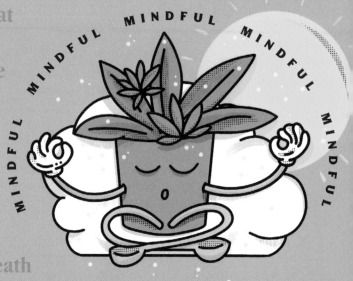

MINDFUL MINDFUL MINDFUL MINDFUL MINDFUL MINDFUL MINDFUL

Mindful Smokes

Sometimes we smoke because we want to party, and at other times we smoke to relax, reflect, and calm ourselves.

Sometimes we smoke because we want to liven things up a bit and party, and at other times we smoke for the opposite effect—to relax, reflect, take time out from busy lifestyles, or simply to calm ourselves at stressful times.

There's a lot to be gained from combining smoking and meditation: a blissful state of marijuana mindfulness.

As you probably know, these are very similar aims of the practice of meditation, and there's a lot to be gained from combining the two in a blissful state of marijuana mindfulness. Pairing mindfulness with a smoke is also a good way of relaxing yourself into meditation if it's something you've never tried before or you have trouble switching off to get started—and a smooth, steady smoke is the perfect excuse for practicing those inhalations and exhalations! Here are ten basic meditations that anyone can do, which, especially if you follow them in sequence, should give your mind and body a refreshing, soothing pause and reset, and let you make the most of marijuana's most magical properties.

Notice your breath

This is a good opener, slowing down the mind and readying it for a steady, relaxing meditation. Sit comfortably, with your smoke ready but not lit, and both feet flat on the floor. Close your eyes, and simply tune yourself into your breathing. Breathe in through your nose and out through your mouth, slowly and steadily, observing each inhalation and exhalation. Notice the air moving through your body, and observe that no two breaths are exactly the same. Count inhalations and exhalations up to ten, then start again from zero. Repeat a few times until you are feeling still.

Tune in to your surroundings

In the same pose, and still breathing carefully, focus on your surroundings. Notice the sounds that you can hear: the wind, cars, leaves in the trees, birdsong. Hear them come and go without judging. Feel the ground beneath your feet, and how it supports your heel and the ball of your foot. Heed how the seat of your chair holds you. Close your eyes.

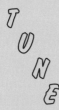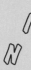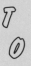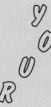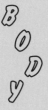

Tune in to your body

Now pay attention to how your body feels. Start with the toes, then work your way through your feet, up your legs, to your torso. Notice any itches, aches, or pains, but don't fight them or judge them: accept them, just as you accept the weight of clothes on your skin or the pulse of blood through your veins. Continue up through the body until you come to the shoulders, then follow your arms down to the fingertips, being aware of all the sensations you encounter along the way. Then back to the shoulders: notice any tension, and the weight of your head, but also feel the strength in your muscles and skeleton. Up through the neck to your head: notice how you hold it, how the skin feels, how your hair and eyebrows touch your face. Continue to the very top of your head, and notice that you feel lighter now, and more grounded. Continue steadily breathing in through your nose, out through your mouth. (Don't try to fight distractions: as other thoughts pop into your mind, observe them, then return to the progress through your body.)

Appreciate what you have

Now open your eyes and let them rest on your joint or pipe. Observe its weight, colors, and smell. Hold it for a moment, noticing how it feels in your hand. Look at it from every angle, and notice the details of its construction, and the way the light falls on it. Run your fingertips over it to feel its texture. Do the same with your lighter or matches. Remember: don't judge—give the lighter the same attention, whether it's made of gold or plastic.

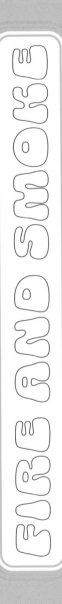

FIRE AND SMOKE

Fire and smoke

Now gently make a flame and look at it for a second—its dark center, its shifting shape and colors, its energy, its warmth. Apply the flame to your joint or pipe, and watch as the fire moves from one to the other, and your grass glows red and starts to smoke. Focus on creating an even, steady glow before you put down the lighter. Be aware of the movement of energy through the leaf, the path of the smoke, and the smell.

Inhalations

Now combine the breath exercises with your joint. Take a few gentle inhalations, and exhale through the nose. Notice the flow of air and smoke through your mouth and into your lungs: its taste, and its temperature. Hold it for an instant, before releasing through your nose. Take as many or as few inhalations as you like, but continue with the careful steady breathing.

Feel the effects

Now return to your body; watch as the weed affects it. Feel your muscles relax, and notice if you feel lighter or heavier, if pains or aches fade. As you did before, continue breathing steadily. Once more, close your eyes, and travel from the base of your feet to your fingertips, and the top of your head.

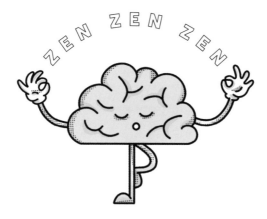

Chants and mantras

You can repeat a phrase over and over again, in time with your breathing. Choose a positive one; as you repeat it, its message will sink gently into your mind. A traditional Hindu mantra is the simplest "Om," which represents the first sound from the beginning of the universe, but also what is now, and what shall be. Close your eyes and repeat it low and slow as you exhale.

Hugs and embraces

If you are smoking and meditating with someone, move to them and exchange a hug. Notice the size and shape of their body, their smell, their breathing, their heartbeat, the feel of their arms around you. Feel the qualities that make them alive and unique. Relax into the embrace and continue breathing mindfully.

Gratitude

By this point you will be profoundly calm and relaxed. Take some time to be grateful: to your body for carrying you, to your loved ones, to the people with you, to the planet for giving you a home, and to the weed which you enjoy. Let your mind wander from one to another, each time thinking of reasons to be thankful. Continue smoking and meditating as long as you want.

Puff and paint
Art appreciation
Free writing
Focused free writing
Marijuana journal
Pot pottery
Liquid light show
Poetry recital
Puff and paint
Art appreciation
Free writing
Focused free writing
Marijuana journal
Pot pottery
Liquid light show
Poetry recital
Puff and paint
Art appreciation
Free writing
Pot pottery
Liquid light show
Poetry recital
Puff and paint
Art appreciation
Free writing
Focused free writing
Marijuana journal

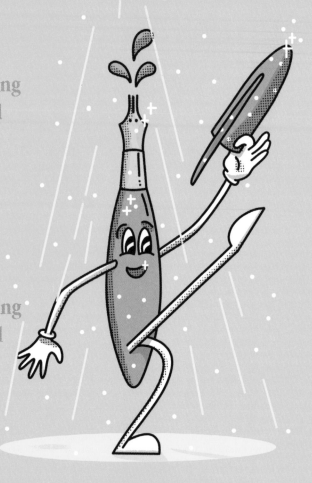

Creative Smokes

It's long been known to psychologists that creativity is an amazing therapy; the simple act of doing something—making something—makes you happy, by putting your mind into a state of "flow," and it also makes you lose track of time, forget about your worries, and enjoy a strong feeling of contentment. Does any of this sound familiar? Marijuana can reduce your inhibitions, improve your confidence, and let your brain make unexpected connections, which can induce you to do some of your best, or at least more experimental, work. So why not combine the two? Have a creative smoke that lets you indulge your endocannabinoid system, and at the same time, let rip your artistic impulses and grant yourself the freedom to express yourself without judgment! Note: this process is also an excellent way of approaching a draft (that's *draft* only…) of that essay or report that's looming over you, which you're just not inspired to write. Let the weed do its work to get those creative juices flowing, then read back in awe later.

It's long been known to psychologists that creativity makes you happy.

Marijuana can reduce your inhibitions, improve your confidence, and let your brain make unexpected connections…

Puff and paint

In weed-oriented vacation destinations like Denver, puff'n'paint studios have become established elements on the tourist trail (see page 91), but there's nothing to stop you from getting going at home. Set up a still life, sit in front of a scenic tree, or persuade a friend to hold a pose for you, and just start drawing or painting as you usually would. Then start on the weed, as you usually would. Use it to relax your eyes, making them more sensitive to perceptions of light, form, and color. It will also reduce your inhibitions, making you more confident with your pencil or brush strokes.

Art appreciation

The beauty of visiting your local art gallery in an altered state is that you get to see familiar works in an entirely new way. You'll obviously need to use edibles, rather than smoke, and that has the advantage of giving you a long, sustained, heavy buzz—perfect for getting sucked into the rich colors of oil paint, appreciating the life in a sculpture, or engaging with the challenge of contemporary conceptual art. Allow yourself plenty of time, take it slow, and let yourself be drawn along by the artists' works.

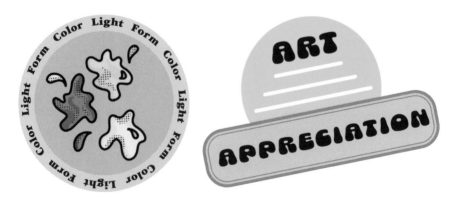

Free Writing...

Free writing

Often used by writers to unblock themselves and also recommended by therapists and teachers, free writing is an excellent way to break down obstacles of low confidence, embarrassment, and fear. Set a timer for ten or fifteen minutes, then pick up a joint with one hand and your pen with the other and just *write*—anything—without regard to topic, spelling, syntax, grammar, or any of the other difficult bits. Don't read your work back as you write and make no corrections. If you can't think of anything to write, write about that; or write about your emotions, physical sensations, or whatever else is on your mind. Go off-topic and let your train of thought travel freely, but write it all down until the alarm sounds. You will be surprised at what you've produced.

Focused free writing

This can be a useful warm-up exercise for students who are intimidated by a looming essay deadline. Once again, pick up your pen and a joint, but this time write freely on the topic in question. This isn't going to be your essay, but it will get your brain moving more confidently around the subject at hand and is an excellent way to sort out your thoughts and brainstorm new ideas and connections.

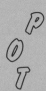

Marijuana journal

Our powers of recall are much less reliable than we would like them to be, yet much of our happiness depends on having good memories at hand when we need an emotional lift. You will remember your days much better if you write about them soon after, and you will remember your highs *much* better if you keep a marijuana journal. Each time you smoke, make a note of how the weed made you feel: the thoughts, perceptions, and laughter that you enjoyed; the taste, smell, circumstances, and people you were with—*everything*. You'll enjoy recalling the smoke at leisure, you'll have a much better memory of it, and at some future date you'll be able to look back and remember the good times in great detail.

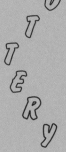

Pot pottery

There is something incredibly... *nice* about the feeling of wet clay in your hands, and even if you don't have a potter's wheel or kiln at home (most of us don't, of course), it's possible to make something attractive and practical using air-drying clay. Pots for your houseplants, ashtrays, and bowls for your munchies are all good starting points; advanced potters may try to make their own clay pipe or bong. Note that smoking a joint while your hands are covered in wet clay can be tricky, so this activity is easier if you've had an edible.

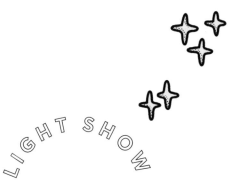

Liquid light show

If you missed the psychedelic scene of 1960s' San Francisco the first time around, don't worry, you can still enjoy the light show today, and the weed is likely to be much better than the stale shwag that most people were smoking back then. First, make friends with a teacher, academic, or school caretaker: you need an old-fashioned overhead projector. (As they upgrade to digital whiteboards, many schools are junking these, so you may get lucky and be able to keep it.) In a darkened room, with some good music on, point the projector at a white wall. Place a clear plastic dish on the projector (the front of an old clock can work well, or a large petri dish). Pour in a couple of tablespoons of water, the same amount of mineral oil (from a drugstore or pharmacy). Add drops of oil-based paint, or ink, and start mixing and adding color!

Poetry recital

You need some like-minded friends for this. Prepare yourselves by picking a poem, practice reading it in front of the mirror (record yourself on your phone, if you really want to work on your delivery), and later, when everyone is good and high, make like you're in a New York coffeehouse back in the 1950s—dress like a Beatnik and perform your verses for everyone else.

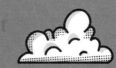

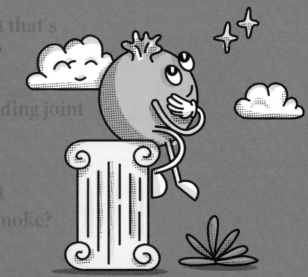

Zeno's arrow
Atalanta's neverending joint
Eubulides stash
Theseus' bong
Can God roll a joint that's
   too big to smoke?
Zeno's arrow
Atalanta's neverending joint
Eubulides stash
Theseus' bong
Can God roll a joint
   that's too big to smoke?
Zeno's arrow

Mind-Blowing Philosophical Paradox Smokes

Eubulides stash
Theseus' bong
Zeno's arrow
Eubulides stash
Theseus' bong
Can God roll a joint
   that's too big to smoke?
Atalanta's neverending joint

We all know that it's possible to have incredible insights into life, the universe, and everything when we are enjoying a reefer or two—although it's sometimes hard to remember these astute comments afterward to regale

Cannabis users have been enjoying enlightening perceptions for thousands of years.

your friends with, or indeed work out exactly what it was that made them seem so incredible at the time. And of course, you aren't the first smoker to experience this conundrum. Cannabis users have been enjoying these enlightening perceptions for thousands of years—certainly back to the time of the ancient Greeks—and have mostly benefitted from them. The profound philosophical musings of such classical scholars might well have been inspired by a toke or a cup of "happy" wine, too. With that idea in mind, here are five of the great philosophers' most intriguing paradoxes—reimagined into stories that, frankly, would have made school a lot more interesting and memorable, and which are guaranteed to blow your mind. Marijuana works its magic in some of the greatest myths here, sorting the possible from the impossible.

We all know that it's possible to have incredible insights into life, the universe, and everything when we are enjoying a reefer or two.

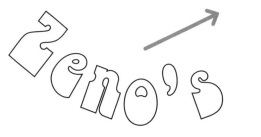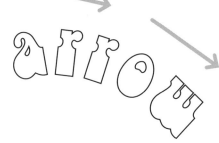

ZENO'S ARROW

Zeno was fond of getting high and shooting arrows from his bow. "Whoa…" said young Socrates. "That's dangerous!" Zeno handed him a joint and pointed to an arrow lying on the ground. "Is this arrow dangerous?" he asked. "No, of course not," said Socrates. "It's not moving."

"Well then, neither is this one," said Zeno, firing an arrow high into the air.

"How do you figure that?" said Socrates, anxiously.

"In a single moment of time, no time passes. The arrow on the ground doesn't move, and in that same instant, neither does the arrow in the air."

"Right…"

"Time is nothing more than a series of moments, right? Yet in that moment, zero motion happens. And in the next moment, and the next. So, that arrow's not moving."

"But…" said Socrates, his mind blown by the paradox and the weed.

"Believe me, kiddo," said Zeno. "Motion is impossible." And he took back the joint and walked away.

AtALANtA'S NeVeReNDING J°INt

Aristotle and the huntress Atalanta were enjoying one last joint at the end of the day. It was the last of their stash: "But don't worry," said Aristotle. "We can make it last forever."

"How?" replied Atalanta.

"It's easy," said Aristotle. "First, you smoke half of the joint, then I smoke half of what's left. Then you smoke half of what's left after that, and we carry on passing it back and forth."

Atalanta complied, and as both she and Aristotle took great care not to smoke more than half of the rest of the joint, they never actually finished it. In fact, they are smoking it to this day, taking ever-smaller puffs, to be sure, but not quite reaching the end.

MIND-BLOWING PHILOSOPHICAL PARADOX SMOKES

tHeseUS' B°NG

The great hero Theseus was an enthusiastic smoker, too, favoring a water pipe on his voyages. Once, while he was at sea, his bong's bowl got gummed up and needed replacing. The mouthpiece soon followed, as did its leather tube, and finally the clay amphora that held the water was cracked and had to be switched out. On Theseus' return to port, Heraclitus, the philosopher, asked if Theseus' bong was the same as the one he'd left with.

"Yes," said Theseus.

"How can it be?" asked Heraclitus. "Everything's changed."

According to Plato, Heraclitus also suggested that it was impossible to step into the same river twice, because the waters were always shifting. Is Theseus' bong an example of an ever-changing river?

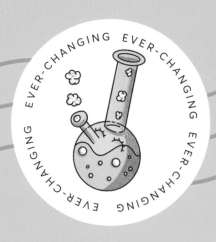

CAN G⁰D R⁰LL A J⁰INt tHAt'S t⁰⁰ BIG t⁰ SM⁰Ке?

Many years later, theologians would wrestle with an even bigger question. If God exists, he must be omnipotent, correct? More powerful than any other being or force in the universe, he would be able to lift any weight, burst from any jail cell, or roll a joint of infinite size. It also stands to reason that he could create anything: a boulder that was too heavy for him to lift, a jail cell that was infinitely strong, or a spliff that was so incredibly loaded with skunk that even a deity would be forced to put it down for a pause. But if he could make that joint (or boulder, or jail cell), then he would be beaten by it. So he wouldn't be omnipotent after all.

EUBULIDES StASH

The philosopher Euclid was a keen home-grower who produced far more than he could actually smoke. He kept a heap of dried buds in his house in Miletus, and one day his student Eubulides came around to bum one for a smoke.

"No problem, man," said Euclid. "I've still got a heap left."

"So you have," replied Eubulides. "Taking one bud away hasn't made any difference—you still have a heap. And if I take another bud away, you will still have a heap. And so on… but at some point, your heap will become a nonheap. But how can it, if one heap minus one bud is still a heap of buds?"

Dennis Peron
Keith Stroup
Jack Herer
Tom Forçade
Steve DeAngelo
Willie Nelson
Ethan Nadelmann
Louis Armstrong
Allen Ginsberg
Brownie Mary
Dennis Peron
Keith Stroup
Jack Herer
Tom Forçade
Steve DeAngelo
Willie Nelson
Ethan Nadelmann
Louis Armstrong
Allen Ginsberg
Brownie Mary
Dennis Peron
Keith Stroup
Jack Herer
Tom Forçade
Steve DeAngelo
Willie Nelson
Ethan Nadelmann

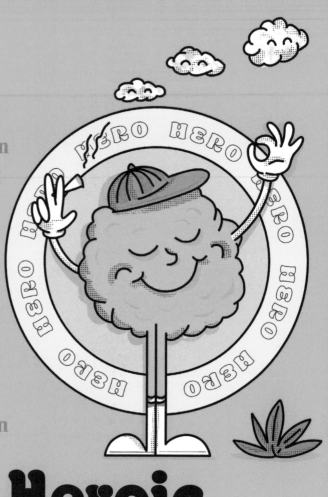

Heroic Smokers

Those who've made it possible.
Those who love the herb.
Those who fight to make it accessible.

Sometimes it's enough simply to relax and enjoy the many benefits of our smoke. The mellow high, the sociability, the way the cares of the day just seem to ease away… it's all good. We shouldn't forget, though, to honor those who've made it possible for us to enjoy this gift—those whose love for the herb led them not simply to enjoy it, but also to fight to make it accessible to the rest of us. Cannabis legalization has been tightly linked to debates around law enforcement and justice, race and economics. Some of these trailblazing smokers not only made cannabis cool and changed the cultural landscape, they also proved

We shouldn't forget to honor those who've made it possible for us to enjoy this gift.

its important medicinal qualities, offering respite from pain for so many, without fear of prosecution. So next time you're rolling a fat one, take a moment to thank these heroic smokers and activists and take steps to support their organizations, whose job is not yet done and who are pressing for more progress and more justice, for tokers the world over.

Louis Armstrong

Louis Armstrong

"We always looked at pot as a sort of medicine, a cheap drunk and with much better thoughts than one that's full of liquor."

It's hard to overstate the contribution of Louis Armstrong to our culture—even if you don't listen to jazz, the music that you do listen to owes him a lot. Not only was his trumpet-playing revolutionary—he invented the solo, as we know it—he was one of the first African–American artists to achieve worldwide fame and respect, and the first popular entertainer to sing in his own voice. If you find operatic vocals artificial and contrived, yet love Bob Dylan, Mick Jagger, Missy Elliott, or Kanye, you should thank Louis, who stepped in front of a microphone and sang the way he spoke. And he *really* loved pot, speaking about it publicly, and warmly, despite the very real risk of legal persecution. Legend has it that when Armstrong met Vice President Nixon at an airport in 1953, the politician politely offered to carry his bag to the plane. It contained three pounds of weed.

Allen Ginsberg

Allen Ginsberg

"What it finally boils down to is that the fear is not about the drugs but about the police."

Allen Ginsberg is primarily remembered now for his poetry, his political radicalism, and his associations with other great creatives like Jack Kerouac and Bob Dylan. Unlike them, though, he was a dedicated activist, who put his money where his mouth was. He wrote convincingly about pot's potential for emotional, spiritual, and artistic development, he campaigned for the release of those locked up for smoking it, and he publicly debated legalization. Much of his writing on the subject went unpublished (an editor at the *New York Times* actually apologized for not having taken his work seriously enough), but some made it into print, and it's great stuff. In *The Great Marijuana Hoax*, he wrote: "Marijuana is a useful catalyst for specific optical and aural aesthetic perceptions... I apprehended the structure of certain pieces of jazz & classical music in a new manner under the influence of marijuana, and these apprehensions have remained valid in years of normal consciousness... And I saw anew many of nature's panoramas & landscapes that I'd stared at blindly without even noticing before; thru the use of marijuana, awe & detail were made conscious." Inspiring words to remember, next time you light up.

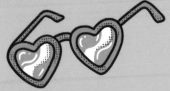

Brownie Mary

Brownie Mary

"My kids need this and I'm ready to go to jail for my principles… I'm not going to cut any deals with them. If I go to jail, I go to jail."

Mary Jane Rathbun was a middle-aged San Francisco waitress when, in 1974, she met Dennis Peron and started making hash brownies. This was an excellent way to make some cash, and by the time of her first bust in 1980, she was baking about 600 a day, and selling most of them to the Castro Street gay community. It was being busted that changed her life, for she was sentenced to community service, which meant that she was volunteering for a community project when the AIDS crisis struck. Rathbun discovered that her brownies helped prevent the physical wasting that AIDS caused, then she found that it also worked for cancer patients undergoing chemo. She started baking huge quantities to help out. Although she was caring for hundreds of sick people, whom she called her "kids" (her own daughter had died in a car crash), Rathbun was prosecuted twice more for possession, each time using her trial to promote the causes of AIDS care and of marijuana as a therapy. It was as a direct result of her efforts that California legalized medical marijuana—a key moment in the journey toward legality that we are now on.

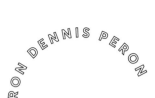

Dennis Peron

"Every cannabis user is a medical patient whether they know it or not."

Brownie Mary did not work alone. Her business partner in the San Francisco Buyers Club was Vietnam veteran Dennis Peron. He had seen how effective cannabis was at easing the symptoms of his partner, Jonathan West, who died of AIDS. In the face of multiple raids from law enforcement, Peron coauthored California Proposition 215, the legislation that permitted medical use of cannabis for compassionate reasons. (He subsequently opposed Propositions 19 and 64, which allowed recreational use, as he believed that all smoking was medicinal.) After standing as a presidential candidate for the Grassroots-Legalize Cannabis Party in 1996 (winning 5,000 votes), he bought a twenty-acre cannabis farm in Northern California and operated it until his death in 2018.

Keith Stroup

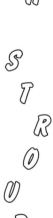

"It should be of no interest or concern to the government. They have no business knowing whether we smoke or why we smoke."

An advocate and activist since the early 1970s, Stroup founded NORML, the National Organization for the Reform of the Marijuana Laws, in 1970. In the decades since, he has been the primary spokesperson for America's marijuana smokers, creating classic ad campaigns, lobbying state and federal government, and—eventually—seeing the tide turn in favor of legalization.

jack herer

Jack Herer

"The only dead bodies from marijuana are in the prisons and at the hands of the police. This is ridiculous."

Some activists—like Stroup—dress respectably and groom conventionally, reasoning that this is how those in power will take you seriously. Not Jack Herer, the self-styled "Hemperor" who looked like the missing Fabulous Furry Freak Brother. Head-shop owner, perennial attention-seeker, and author of the legalization classic *The Emperor Wears No Clothes*, Jack Herer was truly committed to the cause right to the end, suffering a heart attack backstage at a hemp festival in Oregon. A world-beating strain of weed is named after him.

Tom Forçade

"Everything is better with a bag of weed."

Tom Forçade died young but packed plenty into his short life. He got his start in smuggling in the 1960s, throwing bags of weed over remote spots of the Mexican border fence, then tearing around through a border crossing point to pick up the bag on the other side. Never quite abandoning smuggling, he diversified into media, working with the Underground Press Syndicate (which distributed counterculture magazines), and then, in 1974, founded *High Times* magazine, the home of stoner culture to this day. Each issue includes a centerfold of a particularly attractive marijuana plant. The magazine was hugely successful, but Forçade was not able to enjoy the benefits. He blew one fortune on buying racehorses, another on an abortive movie project, and reputedly lost a third when a twenty-ton shipment of grass was intercepted at Jamaica Bay in New York. He killed himself a few days later, at the age of only thirty-three.

Tom Forçade

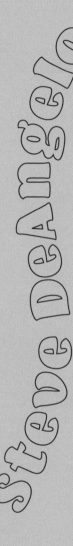

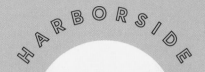

Health Center

- OAKLAND -

Steve DeAngelo

"Defining cannabis consumption as elective recreation ignores fundamental human biology and history, and devalues the very real benefits the plant provides."

Another of the rich crop of medical-marijuana activists that drove a legal and cultural shift in California and then across the U.S., Steve DeAngelo helped Jack Herer publish *The Emperor Wears No Clothes*, started up a number of hemp-related businesses in the 1970s and '80s, and wrote his own book, *The Cannabis Manifesto: A New Paradigm for Wellness*. His most significant move, however, was opening the Harborside Health Center in 2006. This nonprofit dispensary in Oakland eventually gained more than 300,000 registered medical patients and sold the weed for California's first legal recreational joint in 2018. The entrepreneurial DeAngelo expanded his weed empire and now runs Arcview Group, the first commercial cannabis investment fund, which has more than $200 million under management. As if that wasn't enough, in 2019 he founded the Last Prisoner Project, a nonprofit dedicated to the release of all those jailed for marijuana offenses.

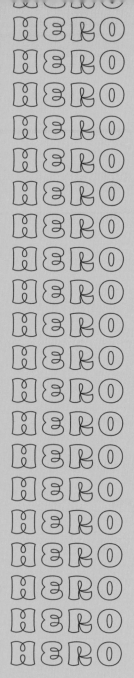

Willie Nelson

"It's nice to watch it being accepted—knowing you were right all the time about it: that it was not a killer drug."

Sheer longevity would make Willie Nelson a poster boy for weed's benefits. At eighty-six, even though emphysema means he can't smoke joints anymore, he's high all day long, thanks to a vaporizer and his side hustle as Chief Tasting Officer of Willie's Reserve, the family cannabis product company. He credits weed for his long life—he gave up drinking and cigarettes in 1978 and found that he was a much nicer, and healthier, person as a result. Despite multiple busts, Willie continued publicly advocating for weed, extolling its economic potential, and campaigning on behalf of jailed victims of punitive anti-drug laws. And he's even smoked a joint on the roof of the White House.

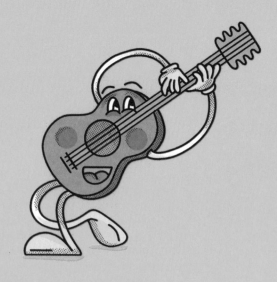

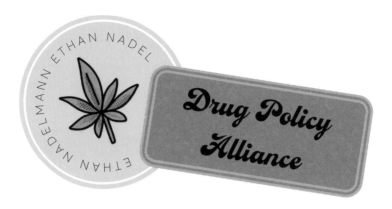

Ethan Nadelmann

"The worst prohibition, it must be said, is a prohibition on thinking—and that, sadly, is what the U.S. government is guilty of today."

The son of a New York rabbi, Nadelmann didn't come to drug reform from a head shop or a Grateful Dead gig, but Harvard, where he started work on his Ph.D. in the 1980s. Looking into the internationalization of crime, he interviewed so many DEA agents that he wound up with a security clearance and a role at the State Department's narcotics bureau. He was not, however, a fan of the "War on Drugs"—his research persuaded him that law enforcement was doing more harm than good. With the support of George Soros, he started the Lindesmith Center, and then the Drug Policy Alliance, campaigning for the legalization of medical marijuana, sentencing reform, and treatment as an alternative to incarceration. More convincing to lawmakers in Washington than California's stable of reformers, Nadelmann has seen steady change and deserves credit for saving lives, reducing incarcerations, and changing attitudes nationally and internationally.

Pain relief
Anti-inflammatory
Weight loss
Regulate diabetes
Stimulate appetite
Improved fracture recovery
Treat depression
Help your mood
Calm your nerves
Treat anxiety
Regulate
  seizures
Better sleep
Pain relief
Anti-inflammatory
Weight loss
Regulate diabetes

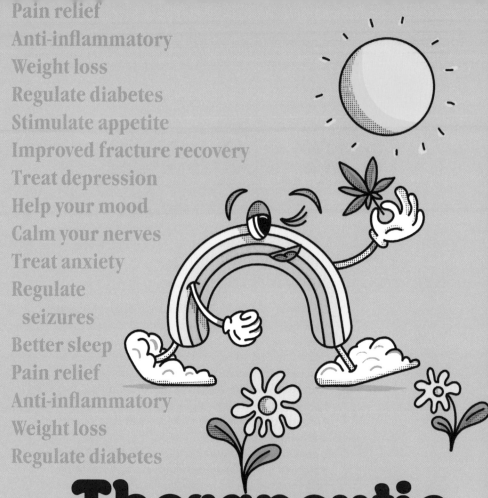

Therapeutic
Smokes

Stimulate appetite
Improved
  fracture recovery
Treat depression
Help your mood
Calm your nerves
Treat anxiety

Recreational smokers should be grateful to the persistent pioneers of medical marijuana, who, sometimes putting their careers on the line, changed the debate around cannabis, revealing its many benefits to our health. While there is still a lot of research and education ahead (and much of the research referred to here is itself very recent), marijuana is now firmly established in the modern pharmacopoeia, and it's clear that it will only become more important to us in years to come.

Marijuana is now firmly established in the modern pharmacopoeia.

What is it in cannabis that works on our brains and bodies? While there are more than sixty active cannabinoid compounds in the marijuana we smoke, the two most important are $\Delta 9$-tetrahydrocannabinol (what we call THC) and cannabidiol (CBD). THC affects our mood, delivering euphoria—and if you're unlucky, psychosis. Note, by the way, that psychosis in this context doesn't refer to anger but a loss of contact with reality—hearing or seeing things that other people can't (hallucinations) or believing things that aren't true (delusions).

Recreational smokers should be grateful to the persistent pioneers of medical marijuana, who changed the debate around cannabis.

CBD, on the other hand, is not psychoactive itself—it doesn't make you high—and is thought to have antianxiety and possibly antipsychotic effects. You could say that CBD tends to balance out some of the effects of THC, so what a given strain of marijuana does to you depends on the proportions of the THC/CBD mix, and the strength of the dose.

THC is available to doctors in a synthetic form (called Nabilone) or naturally derived extract (called Dronabinol). CBD is widely available without prescription. The other sixty active cannabinoids in your joint are not, yet, so it's fair to say that they can only be accessed by consuming weed in its original form. Plenty of research needs to be done on how these other compounds work alone, in conjunction with each other, or in conjunction with other medication. If you want to try CBD treatment for any of the conditions mentioned in this section, it is available in a tincture and usually applied in small doses under the tongue.

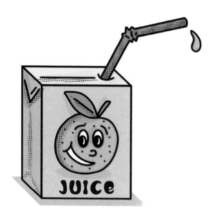

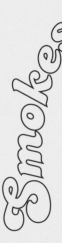

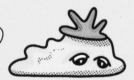

Health risks

You might have heard that marijuana is risk-free—it isn't, but nearly all of the risks apply only with heavy, regular use. In the short term, the effects on memory, judgment, and motor skills make driving very dangerous: *don't do it*; and if you are driving, don't let anyone smoke in your car. Overdosing on THC may result in paranoia, which is highly unpleasant, but will pass. In the long term, smoking weed every day does affect young people's brains—specifically, the amygdala, a part of the brain that deals with emotions and especially fear. This may account for the higher rates of anxiety, depression, and psychotic illness that regular smokers experience. IQ also drops, so remember to take plenty of days off if you're under twenty-five (around which point your brain stops developing). Smoking anything is bad for your throat and lungs, so it also increases the risk of bronchitis, pneumonia, vascular disease, and throat infection. That's the bad news. Now for the good stuff.

Multiple sclerosis

There is strong evidence, from multiple studies, that the pain and spasticity (muscle tightness) of MS can be effectively treated with a combination of THC and CBD. If you are receiving treatment for MS already, your doctor will certainly know about this.

Chronic pain

If you have a pain that won't go away, the THC in marijuana may help, although you should always seek other solutions and professional medical advice as well.

Lung capacity

Smoking weed is always going to be bad for your lungs, and it increases the risk of a variety of respiratory illnesses. However, there is research that confirms that CBD administered on its own has anti-inflammatory effects that can, in fact, improve lung function and help fight some respiratory diseases.

Lose weight

Yes, you read that right. Marijuana famously encourages us to sit on a sofa and eat unhealthy food, but that is a function of the THC in your smoke. CBD, on the other hand, has several effects on the body that may help you to lose weight. To start with, anecdotal evidence, plus animal tests, suggest that it may suppress appetite, so you feel less of an urge to eat. Then a 2016 study found that CBD stimulates the production (in your cells) of several proteins that turn "white" fat into "brown" fat—which is healthier. This same process may also burn off calories, giving yet another benefit.

Regulate diabetes

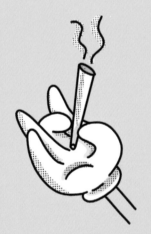

There is evidence that CBD, in conjunction with another cannabinoid with the catchy name of tetrahydrocannabivarin, lowered blood sugar levels and increased insulin production in patients with type 2 diabetes. Tetrahydrocannabivarin is also known as THCV and is not a controlled substance in the U.S.

Cancer

One common side-effect of cancer treatments is that they cause the patient to lose their appetite. This is one area when THC's appetite stimulation comes into its own.

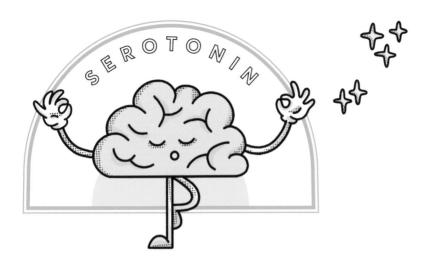

Depression

CBD has an effect on serotonin receptors in the brain. Serotonin is one of the hormones of happiness and low stress, so low serotonin levels are probably connected to depression. On its own, CBD doesn't stimulate serotonin production, but by affecting how your brain's chemical receptors react to the serotonin that your body naturally makes, it can help your mood. Studies in 2014 and 2018 showed that CBD has antidepressant and antistress qualities.

Anxiety

For similar reasons, CBD seems to help with anxiety, too—so the next time you're nervous about making a public appearance, or you're trying to focus for an exam, consider using a little.

Regulating seizures

There is good evidence to show that some forms of epilepsy (specifically, Dravet and Lennox-Gastaut Syndromes) may be alleviated by CBD. Better research in this area is urgently needed as many existing seizure medications have strong, undesirable side effects that CBD avoids.

Fracture recovery time

In 2018, the *Journal of Bone and Mineral Research* published a study demonstrating that CBD not only accelerates the healing of bone fractures, but also leaves the healed bone stronger than it was before.

Glaucoma

Cannabis may help a little with this eye condition, but it isn't a miracle cure. It was first reported in 1971 that THC's blood-pressure-reducing properties would help patients with glaucoma (an eye condition caused by high pressure in the eye), but two big problems make it an impractical therapy. Firstly, CBD will tend to have the opposite effect, increasing pressure in the eye, so smoking a joint with both THC and CBD cannabinoids in it will tend not to do much. Secondly, if you can apply THC alone, then it needs to be used continuously… meaning that you would have to be high all the time.

Alzheimer's and dementia

Neither CBD nor THC can stop or slow down the brain diseases that lead to dementia; they can, though, help with some of the symptoms, which often include anxiety, agitation, or anger.

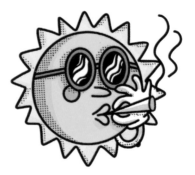

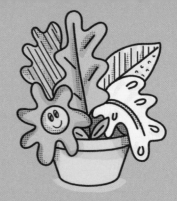

Arthritis pain

Laboratory studies on animals suggest CBD's pain-relieving and anti-inflammatory properties work on the symptoms of arthritis, but these effects haven't (yet) been validated in large-scale human testing. That said, unsurprisingly, some arthritis suffers who have tried CBD report noticeable pain relief, less anxiety, and better sleep—so it may be worth a try.

Hepatitis C

A 2017 study by Jamaican doctors revealed that CBD may be effective in inhibiting this serious viral infection. While it has not yet been approved for use, it seems likely to form the basis of a therapy at some point in the future.

IBS

Cannabinoid receptors are found throughout the body, not just in the brain, and CBD has a beneficial effect on many of the symptoms of IBS and related digestive disorders. Anecdotal evidence suggests that these can be dramatic.

Parkinson's disease

Multiple studies show that CBD has benefits across a wide range of symptoms of Parkinson's disease: tremors, psychosis, sleep problems, depression, anxiety, and pain. Some researchers report great improvements in patients' quality of life, with no side-effects, making this a valuable addition to the available therapies.

Banana bong
Make your own hashish
The hot roll method
The frying pan method
Hand-rolled in the wild
Liquid vaping
Dry herb vaping
One-hitter
Dabbing
Hot knives
Bucket bong
Pool bong
Hookah
Blunt
Carve your own pipe
Banana bong
Make your own hashish
The hot roll method
The frying pan method
Hand-rolled in the wild
Liquid vaping
Dry herb vaping
One-hitter
Dabbing
Hot knives
Bucket bong
Pool bong

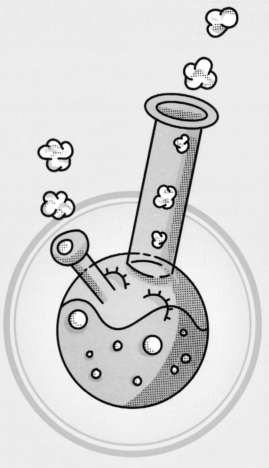

Tips & Tricks

Smoking is a simple principle, with many interesting spins. There are *so* many more ways to administer the herb than simply skinning up, and the smoke will hit you in a fascinatingly varied way with each different mode you try. Be inspired to vape, dab, and bucket your way to interesting new highs, or experiment with hookahs, buckets, and more; then impress your friends with lucid critiques of the fine and subtle variations between each one. Or, maybe, just enjoy the mellow.

There are so many more ways to administer the herb than simply skinning up.

If you're into smoking you're probably into the little knick-knacks that go along with the habit—especially pipes. Head shops are fun places to hang out and shop in, but it's really much more satisfying to make your own paraphernalia. It's also useful to know how to turn the dust in the bottom of your grinder into portable, long-lasting, smooth-smoking hashish…

Be inspired to vape, dab, and bucket your way to interesting new highs, or experiment with hookahs, buckets, and more.

Techniques

Liquid vaping

Ideal for the health conscious, or anyone smoking marijuana medicinally, vaping liquids is much better for you (less crud into your lungs), more comfortable (no more coughing fits), and more efficient (less of the THC and CBD get burned off or lost in the smoke). It's more discreet, too. However, it can be hard to source vape oil with THC in it, and you lose all of those connoisseur's pleasures to do with aroma, strain, taste, and appearance.

Dry herb vaping

If you want to retain those aspects of the smoke, try a conduction or convection vaper. These don't need liquids but will instead heat dry herb to the point that it releases the THC, CBD, and terpenes without sparking a flame. These are discreet, easy to manage, and you can use them with your regular stash. Many models now come with a temperature gauge so you can cook your bud exactly the way you like it.

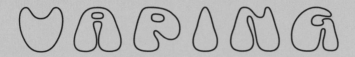

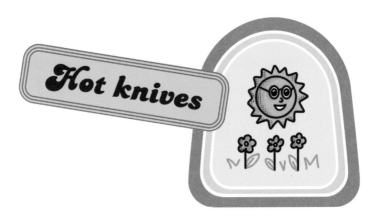

One-hitter

A one-hitter is perfect if you like to hit it and quit it, taking a good draw and carrying on with your day. You don't ignite the weed, instead warming the small bowl that it sits in, so (like a dry herb vape) you get all of the good stuff and none of the carcinogenic crud that you get from burning leaves and stems. Less useful, perhaps, if you want a heavy couch session and don't want to have to refill every time you take a hit.

Hot knives

Of all the ways to enjoy cannabis, this—sometimes known as spotting—is perhaps the low down and dirtiest. First, cut a large plastic drink bottle in half. Hold the top half (the spout) in your mouth with your teeth. Then take two regular kitchen knives and heat the tips of their blades over the stove (a gas stove is best for this, but electric burners do the job, too). When they are seriously hot (maybe not red hot, but getting there), grip a small lump of hash, or bud, between them. It will start to smoke—inhale the smoke through the bottle. This is a fun trick for parties, with an enjoyable whiff of danger, but it's hardly sophisticated.

Dabbing

If you've got some hash oil, dabbing with a waterpipe is the way to go. Many connoisseurs swear by the dab: by heating the oil until it smokes, you produce a concentrated, potent vapor, and by bubbling it through water, you cool it so it's comfortable to inhale deeply.

Hookah

If you don't mind a little ostentation in your home, a traditional Middle Eastern hookah (or hubbly-bubbly) is a sociable way to smoke. For best results, mix the weed with some shisha tobacco, fire up the coals, and pass the mouthpiece around the circle of a few friends.

Blunt

While a joint may be a practical everyday solution to your smoking needs, there's something to be said for taking the time and trouble to make yourself a nice, fat, traditional, hip-hop style blunt. The tobacco in the leaf adds its distinctive edge to your high, the smoke can taste luxurious (especially if you use an upmarket cigar for your wrap), and blunts are big, slow burners, making them ideal for sharing with a close friend or two. Split a fresh cigar or cigarillo down its length, moisten the wrapper lightly to make it easier to work, fill it with weed (more than you would use in a joint), roll it, lick it, smooth it shut. It will still be a little moist, so warm it lightly with a flame to dry it out before smoking. Enjoy!

ROLL IT

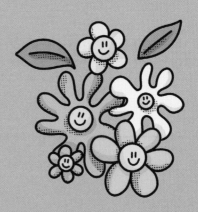

Bucket bong

If you've tried the hot knives technique, you'll have half of a plastic drink bottle on hand. Take a clean bucket and fill it with water. Take a small piece of tinfoil and make lots of tiny holes in it with the point of a sharp pencil, then fit the foil into the mouthpiece of the bottle so it forms a concave bowl. Put some weed or hash into this bowl, then gently lower the bottle into the bucket so the water is just underneath the level of the spout. Heat the cannabis with a lighter, and as it starts to burn, pull the bottle up slowly so that it fills with smoke, trapped by the water in the bucket. Take the foil off the top, place your lips over the mouth of the bottle, and inhale deeply at the same time as pushing your head (and the bottle) downward. You will end up with two lungs full of fresh hash vapor. Success!

Pool bong

Like a bucket bong, except that you use your pool for a bucket. Do this in the shallow end and do not attempt to swim when high!

Manufactory

Carve Carve Carve Carve Carve Carve

Carve your own pipe

There's something much more relaxing about the time-honored practice of smoking a pipe rather than a joint. After all, it's the way we did it for thousands of years, before the cigarette paper arrived in the second half of the nineteenth century.

It's easy to make a basic pipe with just a block of hardwood—about 1 x 1 x 4 inches—and a hand drill. (You can even use a tree branch if it's not green wood, but has been allowed to season and dry out.) Use a ½-inch bit to drill out a bowl, about ¾ inch deep, near one end of one of the long surfaces of the wood. Then use a ¼-inch bit to drill a narrower hole in the center of the smaller surface at the far end of the pipe. This hole will go straight down the center of the block to the bottom of the bowl. *Voilà!* You can use this right away to smoke.

A pipe filter (a small metal mesh that you can find at a head shop or vape store) placed in the bottom of the bowl will give you a smoother burn. Once you've tested the pipe, you can carve, whittle, saw, or sand the outside of the block to whatever shape you like, keep it as a minimalist cuboid, or whittle around your bowl and mouthpiece to produce something truly unique.

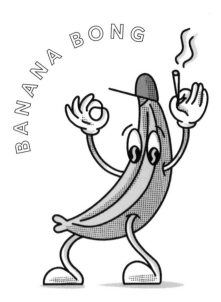

Banana bong

This is the lowest-budget pipe of them all—and yet the most nutritious. You need a banana—preferably still a little green—a knife, and a ballpoint pen. Slice off the tip of the banana (the far end from the stem). You want to take at least 1½ inches off—this will form the bowl of the pipe. Cut the very tip off this piece (the last ¼ inch) so that it has a flat base. Scoop out the fruit and eat it. Yum. The bowl should have a small hole at the bottom. If it doesn't, no problem, press through with the pen to make a hole. Now go back to the banana: stick your pen into the open end to make a tube for the smoke. Go right down the middle, as far as the bend in the banana will allow. Then make another hole to meet it, on the top of the banana, through the peel. Blow through it to ensure that the holes connect and there is a good air flow (you may have to suck out some tasty mushed banana). Use the tip of the knife to open out this second hole so that the bowl will sit neatly in it. Fill the bowl with bud, light it up, and inhale at the end of the banana. Cool, fruity, cooling, fruit.

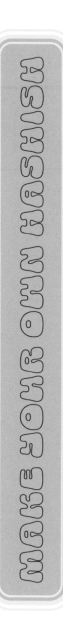

Make your own hashish—the hot roll method

The bud of the plant isn't the only place to find the good stuff: tiny growths called trichomes, rich in cannabinoids, are found on the rest of the greenery. These potent fragments fall off when you freeze the plant (so industrial hashish-making uses dry ice and filters to extract them). You can collect them easily at home if you have a three-part grinder (available from a head shop) that collects the tiny trichomes—they will look like a fine green dust—in a trim bin in its base.

It's possible to make hash resin from these with heat and pressure. One way is to collect the trichomes (or *kief*, to give it its traditional name) in a roasting bag, then roll them flat using a wine bottle full of hot water, pressing hard. When you have squashed the trichomes into a flat piece, fold it back on itself and roll again. Repeat (many times) until you have a block of smooth crumbly resin. This will keep for a long time and not be as smelly as bud.

Make your own hashish—the frying pan method

An alternative is to warm a couple of tablespoons of dry *kief* in a pile in the middle of a clean frying pan, over a low heat. To one side of the pan, put a drop of water; when this starts to boil off, quickly take the pan off the heat. Add a couple of drops of water to the pile of warm *kief*—just enough to make the powder clump together. Mix with a teaspoon, then carefully pick it out of the pan and roll the damp mixture between your palms until it forms a ball. Use the ball to pick up any remnants of *kief* in the pan.

Make your own hashish—hand-rolled in the wild

If you're lucky enough to have many fresh cannabis plants on hand, then you can make your own hash by rolling the buds gently between your palms. (This can be very useful in the field, as it means that you don't have to cure the leaf and you can enjoy the benefit there and then.) Make sure that your hands are clean, and don't apply moisturizer! The trichomes, or *kief*, will coat your hands with sticky resin as you rub the buds. With firm dabs of your thumb you can slowly collect a lump of hash out of the resin on your hands, rolling it as you go. Be patient—it takes a while—but you will end up with a good-sized lump that's ready for immediate use. This method is traditional in the Indian subcontinent and Jamaica, and is likely one of the oldest ways there is to extract cannabis from the cannabis plant.

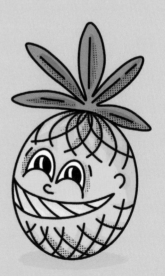

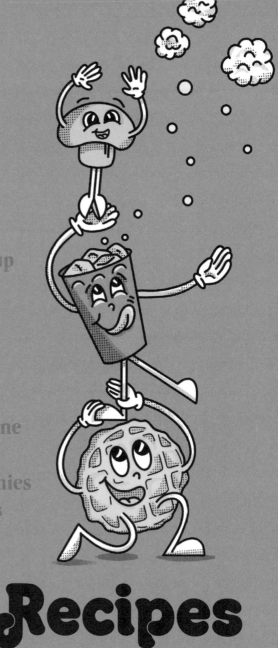

Recipes

There is nothing quite as potent as an edible, and no friendlier gift for a fellow stoner than a tasty little something...

Here are 42.0 ways for you to get your buzz on in the kitchen!

Smoking is by its nature an inefficient business: every toke you take flames off a bit of the good stuff, and many people don't enjoy inhaling burning vegetation. But don't let these two excellent arguments against smoking stop you from trying the magic of marijuana; if you're not fond of a puff, try eating your bud instead. There is nothing quite as potent as an edible, and no friendlier gift for a fellow stoner than a tasty little something that also has a little bit of happiness baked into it, so here are 42.0 ways for you to get your buzz on in the kitchen! We'll start with the basics—showing you how to pull the precious THC and CBD out of the bud and into an ingredient—then move on to how you can build up a stockpile of essentials that you can use to give every dish a little kick, before introducing you to mind-bending main meals, drinks to soothe, to chill out or get the party started with, as well as delicious treats for a post-gym cooldown or an amazing afternoon tea. There's something for every occasion—although perhaps not for the school bake sale…

Go Low, Start Slow

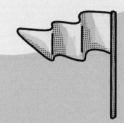

The dosages below, estimated using the potency calculator at loudbowl.com, are approximate and assume that your bud has a THC content of about 15 percent. Your dispensary will be able to tell you more about the potency of the weed you use. You should always err on the side of caution when cooking with cannabis products: if it's too weak, it doesn't matter much. Just consume a little more and make it stronger next time.

Overdoing it on an edible can be unpleasant! You may experience some anxiety or nausea, and it takes a while for the symptoms to pass. Or you may just fall asleep and miss out on all the fun. In any case, take care not to put too much "happy" ingredient into your cooking, and once you've consumed it, give your buzz plenty of time to arrive. Don't assume that you need another brownie after twenty minutes; it can take up to two hours for the effects of an edible to kick in.

A microdose of THC is about 1–2.5 milligrams: a good place for first-timers to start. At the other end of the scale, 25–30 milligrams of THC will have a strong effect, even on someone who uses cannabis a lot. Your coordination and judgment will be affected and you'll be euphoric, but if you're not used to it, you run the risk of nausea and other unpleasant side-effects. Portion control in these recipes is based on a cautious 5 milligrams per portion, but this is an approximate estimate; the actual concentration may vary according to the strength of your bud, the success of the infusion, and so on.

As a rule of thumb, a quarter-ounce of decarboxylized bud contains about 1 gram of THC. That's 200 basic portions—so a little goes a long way!

Condiments & Infusions

Your essential stockpile of ingredients to make any meal "happy," whether served on the side or used as an essential part of the recipes that follow.

Cannabis oil

A 16 fluid ounce bottle of cannabis oil may contain about 1 gram of THC.

A small amount—half a teaspoon—is about one low dose.

Any of the oils that you like to cook with (olive, sunflower, canola) can be made into cannabis oil. If you want to make mayonnaise with it, I recommend light-tasting sunflower oil; if you want to use it for salad dressings, go with an olive oil instead.

¼ ounce **weed**

2 cups **vegetable oil**

Paper coffee filters and **pour-over coffee maker**

1. First you need to decarboxylize your weed, which converts the THCA found in dried buds to THC.

2. Warm the vegetable oil in a medium pan over low heat. While it's warming up, grind your bud.

3. Add the bud to the oil and stir it through. Leave the heat on low and let the hot oil infuse with the bud for about 45 minutes, stirring regularly.

4. Switch off the heat and leave to cool. Using a coffee filter and pour-over coffee maker, strain the oil into a jug. Keep the oil in a sealed glass (not plastic) jar for up to 3–4 months for maximum taste and freshness.

Cannabutter

If you enjoy cooking, it's always useful to keep some Cannabutter in the fridge. Any time a recipe calls for basic butter, just add some of this and you've got a happy recipe...

¼ ounce **weed**

4 cups **water**

1 pound **salted or unsalted butter**, cut into chunks

Paper coffee filters and **pour-over coffee maker**

1. First you need to decarboxylize your weed, which converts the THCA found in dried buds to THC. Preheat the oven to 240°F. Grind your bud up nice and fine, then sprinkle it over a baking sheet. Bake in the oven for about 40 minutes until it's crumbly and has gone from light green to light brown.

2. Now heat the water in a medium pan. When it's boiling, take the heat right down to low, place the chunks of butter into the pan and melt them. When the butter is melted, add the bud, and stir it in.

3. With the pan over the lowest heat, cook for about 1 hour 30 minutes. It may simmer, but don't let it boil: add a little more water if necessary. Stir every 10 minutes or so.

4. After 1 hour 30 minutes, switch off the heat. Now you need to filter out the fragments of bud from the butter. Set the paper filter inside the pour-over coffee maker over a jug or bowl, pour in the hot mixture and let it run through the paper. Some butter will be left behind: squish as much as you can through using a spatula or your fingers.

5. Pour the filtered mixture into a flat-bottomed dish and place it in the fridge to set overnight. In the morning, you'll find that the butter will have set on top of a layer of brownish water. The brownish water contains all the crud that you don't want—think of it as culinary bongwater—so scrape it off and toss it down the sink. Keep the butter in the fridge until you're ready to cook with it.

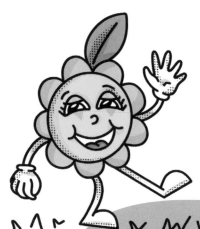

Cannabis vinaigrette

Shake up 4 teaspoons of Cannabis-infused olive oil (see page 175) with about the same amount of white wine vinegar or balsamic vinegar, add a pinch of salt and pepper, and a teaspoon of wholegrain mustard. This will give four salads a modest dose and a distinctive aroma. (If your cannabis oil is particularly strong-smelling, it may not make a pleasant vinaigrette, so taste-test it before you commit yourself.)

Marijuana milk

Use full-fat, or whole, milk for this recipe, rather than skim milk. The milk has a distinctive (instantly recognizable…) flavor, but it will work fine on your cereal or in your coffee.

¼ ounce **weed**

1 pint **milk**

1. First decarboxylize your weed and convert the THCA found in dried buds to THC. Preheat the oven to 240°F. Grind your bud up, then sprinkle it over a baking sheet. Bake in the oven for about 40 minutes until it's crumbly and has gone from light green to light brown.

2. In a small saucepan, over low heat, heat the milk but do not let it simmer or boil. Stir in the decarboxylized weed and let it infuse in the hot milk for 45 minutes, taking care not to let it overheat. After 45 minutes, take the pan off the heat and let it cool, then strain the milk through a sieve over a bowl or jug. Pour the filtered milk into a jar or bottle with a lid and it will keep for up to a week in the fridge.

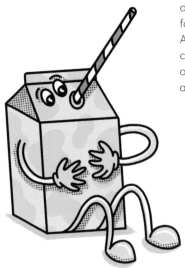

Weed mayonnaise

Cannabis oil makes excellent mayonnaise! This is one of the classic condiments of French cooking, perfect for giving your happy kitchen a little class.

3 **egg yolks** (from the freshest eggs you can find)

½ teaspoon **Dijon mustard**

1 teaspoon **lemon juice**

1 teaspoon **white wine vinegar**

1 cup **homemade Cannabis oil** (made with sunflower oil, see page 175)

Pinch of **salt**, to taste

1. Carefully separate the egg yolks from the whites. In a bowl, use a fork to break the yolks, then whisk in the mustard, lemon juice, and vinegar.

2. Continue whisking as you very slowly add the oil. It should be a very fine stream, allowing the oil and the fat to steadily emulsify together and become thick; use a milk jug to control the amount easily. This stage will take a few minutes.

3. Taste and season. Keep in an airtight glass jar in the fridge and use within 3–4 days.

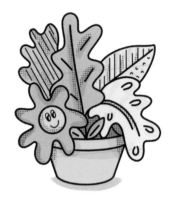

Cannabis "flour"

Another shortcut to happy baking. Note that this "flour" (in fact, more of a spice blend) will definitely taste of marijuana greenery, so you might not want to use too much in the mix.

¼ ounce **weed**

1. First you need to decarboxylize your weed, which converts the THCA found in dried buds to THC. Preheat the oven to 240°F. Pick the stem out of your grass, break up the tender buds, then sprinkle them over a baking sheet. Bake in the oven for about 40 minutes until it's crumbly and has gone from light green to light brown.

2. Using a coffee grinder or food processor, reduce the decarboxylized bud to a fine powder.

3. Keep in an airtight container and use within 3–4 weeks. When baking, use a small amount sprinkled into the flour of your chosen baking recipe.

Cannabis sugar

Mmmm, something nice for your coffee! Or your brownies. Or your muesli.

¼ ounce **weed**

1 cup **vodka**, or similar high-proof clear alcohol

1 cup **white sugar**

1. First you need to decarboxylize your weed, which converts the THCA found in dried buds to THC. Preheat the oven to 240°F. Break up the tender buds, then sprinkle them over a baking sheet. Bake in the oven for about 40 minutes until it's crumbly and has gone from light green to light brown.

2. Stir the buds into the vodka, and let it stand, sealed, in a jar or glass bottle for at least 24 hours. The longer you leave it, the more THC will be dissolved into the vodka, so there's no rush.

3. Preheat the oven to 200°F. Strain the infused vodka into a glass baking dish and discard the old leaf. Add the sugar to the baking dish and mix it thoroughly with the vodka.

4. Bake in the oven for about 20–30 minutes, stirring every 5 minutes, until the alcohol has evaporated and the sugar has taken on a golden color, looking like light brown sugar. Use the sugar as you choose for adding to baking, coffee, or breakfast.

Cannabis coconut oil

A dairy-free, plant-based alternative to Cannabutter (see page 176), you make this in a similar way and use it in a host of different recipes—and skin treatments. It takes longer to infuse and the method is different, though.

¼ ounce **weed**

2 cups **unrefined organic coconut oil**

1. First decarboxylize your weed, to convert the THCA to THC. Preheat the oven to 240°F. Break up the buds, then sprinkle them over a baking sheet. Bake in the oven for about 40 minutes until the leaf is crumbly and has gone from light green to light brown.

2. Mix the coconut oil and the leaf together in a Mason jar and put the lid loosely over the top—don't screw it down. Place the jar in a large saucepan and add water to above the level of oil in the jar. Put a lid on the saucepan and put it on a burner over low heat.

3. Keep the water in the pan simmering for about 4 hours, topping it up as necessary so the water level doesn't drop below the top of the oil.

4. Let the oil cool, then filter it into a fresh sealed jar and keep it in the fridge.

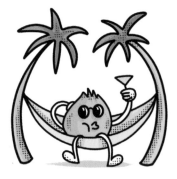

Sustaining Main Meals

Using the condiments and infusions above, it's possible to make a "happy" version of nearly any dish. Here are some ideas to get you going.

MAKES

4

portions

Tomato sauce

A simple tomato sauce for pasta makes an excellent "happy" meal. This recipe makes four portions with modest doses of THC.

4 **garlic cloves**

2 tablespoons **olive oil**

Two 14-ounce cans of **chopped tomatoes**

½ teaspoon **salt**

1 teaspoon **sugar**

A pinch of **dried oregano**

2 teaspoons **Cannabis oil** (see page 175)

1. Finely chop the garlic cloves, then warm the olive oil in a medium saucepan. Add the garlic and fry for a minute but don't let it burn. Add the chopped tomatoes, salt, sugar, and a pinch of dried oregano. Cook with the lid on over gentle heat for 30 minutes.

2. Add the cannabis oil to the sauce as it cooks, stirring it thoroughly.

Canaquesadillas

A simple light lunch that is endlessly flexible.

2 flour tortillas

Your preferred fillings:
refried beans, chopped red onion, grated hard cheese, jalapeños, chopped red bell pepper, chili, sour cream, chives, salsa

½–1 teaspoon **Cannabis oil** (see page 175)

Butter, for frying

1. Use two flour tortillas to sandwich any combination you like of refried beans, chopped red onion, grated hard cheese, jalapeños, chopped red bell pepper, chili, sour cream, chives, or salsa. Drizzle the cannabis oil in with the other fillings.

2. Fry the quesadilla in butter in a frying pan set over medium heat, carefully flipping once, until the filling is piping hot and the tortillas are just starting to crisp up. Eat immediately.

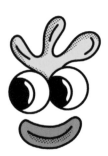

Potato salad

So simple and delicious on a hot day.

½ pound **small potatoes**

1–2 teaspoons
Weed mayonnaise
(see page 179) per person

Chopped scallions
or **red onion**

A drop of **balsamic vinegar**

Wholegrain **mustard**

Boil the potatoes until cooked through, cut them into halves or quarters, let them cool, then mix them up with the mayonnaise, chopped scallions or red onion, a drop of balsamic vinegar, and some wholegrain mustard. Season to taste.

Mushroom omelet

An omelet is simple, quick, cheap, and takes cannabis nicely through oil or butter—sprinkling grass on top of an omelet as though it is an herb will not be effective.

5 **eggs**

A pinch of **salt**

1 teaspoon **Cannabis oil**
(see page 175) or 1 teaspoon
Cannabutter (see page 176)

1 cup **mushrooms**

Break the eggs into a bowl and mix in a pinch of salt and either 1 teaspoon of cannabis oil or 1 teaspoon of cannabutter. Fry some mushrooms in the oil or butter, then cook the omelets one by one, adding half the mushroom on top of each omelet as it solidifies.

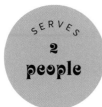

Butternut squash soup

Delicious, healthy, and full of good vibes, Butternut squash soup is wonderfully simple to prepare and perfect for a cozy meal on a cold day.

1 medium **butternut squash**

1 **shallot or onion**

1 **garlic clove**

Butter and olive oil, for frying

1 pint **vegetable broth**

1 teaspoon **Cannabis oil** (see page 175) per portion

1. Preheat the oven to 400°F. To get the richest flavor from your squash, halve it, remove the seeds and skin, and roast it for about 45 minutes in the oven before chopping it into small pieces.

2. Then fry some shallot (or onion) and garlic in butter and olive oil, add the squash pieces and the vegetable broth. You can add more flavor with a sprinkling of ground nutmeg or a tablespoon of maple syrup or sour cream or butter, then add the cannabis oil. Simmer for about 10 minutes, then blend before serving.

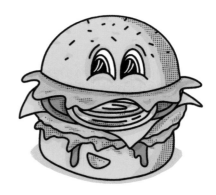

Cannabis burgers

The easiest way to happy up your burger or veggie burger is to add a teaspoon or two of Cannabis mayonnaise (see page 176) to the fillings as you assemble the burger. Alternatively, if you're confident with your dosing and cooking in bulk, you could add Cannabis "flour" (see page 180) to the hamburger mix: dosing this will be easier if you're cooking a large batch at a time. This recipe makes eight quarter-pounder burgers with moderate doses.

¼ batch of **Cannabis flour** (see page 180)

2 pounds **ground beef**

Vegetable oil, for frying

Your favorite burger accompaniments

1. Mix the cannabis flour through the beef. Divide into eight equal patties and press flat.

2. Fry in a hot pan with a splash of vegetable oil to prevent sticking: warm your buns in the oven (set to low) at the same time. Season with salt and pepper after you've browned the patties.

3. Assemble with cheese, ketchup, lettuce leaves, sliced tomato, pickle, sliced red onion…. You need me to tell you what goes into a burger now?

Chili con cannabis

A basic chili of beef, chicken, or vegetables can be improved with the addition of Cannabis oil (see page 175).

1 **onion**, chopped

1 **garlic clove**, chopped

1 **green bell pepper**, deseeded and chopped

Vegetable oil, for frying

1 tsp **chili seasoning mix**, from a packet, or make your own (see tip)

1 teaspoon **Cannabis oil** (see page 175) per portion

1 pound **ground beef or chopped chicken**

One 14-ounce can of **chopped tomatoes**

1 teaspoon **sugar**

1. Fry the onion, garlic, and pepper in vegetable oil, then add some chili seasoning mix and stir through the vegetables for a minute or two. Add the cannabis oil, stirring through so it's evenly distributed.

2. Add the meat and brown for a couple of minutes. Add the chopped tomatoes and the sugar and simmer over low heat, stirring frequently, for 30–40 minutes. Season to taste.

Tip:
To make your own chili seasoning mix, combine 1 tablespoon ground cumin, 1 teaspoon smoked paprika, 1 teaspoon cocoa powder, ½ teaspoon garlic salt, ½ teaspoon onion salt, ½ teaspoon dried red chili flakes, and ½ teaspoon cayenne pepper in a container and seal.

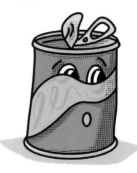

Pasta carbonara

A quick dish that nevertheless offers sensational flavor.

1 ounce smoked **bacon lardons**

4 ounces **spaghetti**

1 **egg yolk**

A dollop of **heavy cream**

Plenty of finely grated **Parmesan**

1 teaspoon **Cannabutter** (see page 176) per portion

A grind of **black pepper**

1. Fry the bacon lardons until they are crispy, then put to one side. Cook the spaghetti in a pan of boiling water according to the packet instructions.

2. While the pasta cooks, mix the egg yolk with a dollop of cream, plenty of finely grated Parmesan, the cannabutter, and a grind of black pepper. Mix the lardons, along with the fat from the pan, into this sauce.

3. When the spaghetti is cooked, drain it and return it to the hot pan, then quickly stir the egg mixture in so that it coats and cooks on the surface of the hot pasta.

Tip:
For a vegetarian version, or just a change, you could substitute chopped mushrooms for the bacon.

Drinks

Mixing your cannabis with a hot drink may make your body absorb it more quickly, so be ready for a faster hit!

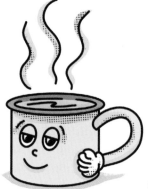

Canna coffee

Make your coffee however you like it (cannalatte, cannacino, flat canna white…), then stir in ½–1 teaspoon of Cannabis sugar (see page 181).

Hot pot chocolate

Heat a couple of tablespoons of water in a pan and dissolve drinking chocolate powder into it (suggested amount is 2 heaped teaspoons per cup, or to taste). Add 10 fluid ounces of milk, then stir in ½–1 teaspoon of Cannabis sugar (see page 181). Heat gently, taking the pan off the heat before the milk boils.

Milkshake

A few scoops of
ice cream, 1 pint of milk,
½–1 teaspoon of Cannabis
sugar (see page 181)… Blend
quickly and drink from a
chilled—very chilled—glass.

Spiced Mary Jane tisane

The classic tisane is an invitation to express
your creativity. Use mint leaves, lime leaves,
finely sliced ginger, and lemongrass; or go
floral with rosehips, lemon verbena,
hibiscus, or camomile. Add the leaves to
a teapot, pour over boiling water, and let
the ingredients infuse for 5 minutes.
Stir ½–1 teaspoon of Cannabis sugar
(see page 181) into your cup.

Happy iced tea

The perfect cooler on a hot summer's day,
iced tea is a fine delivery mechanism for a nice
buzz. Put 4 tea bags into a teapot, pour over
1¾ pints of boiling water, and let it infuse for
5 minutes. Remove the tea bags, pour the tea
into a jug, and stir in 2 tablespoons of sugar,
1 tablespoon of honey, and 1 tablespoon of
Cannabis sugar (see page 181). Stir until
everything is dissolved, then chill in the fridge.
Before serving, add the juice of 2 lemons,
some slices of orange, and a sprig of mint.
Serve in glasses over ice.

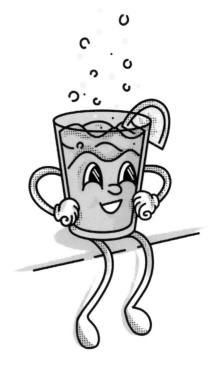

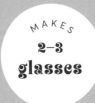

Bhang lassi

This recipe differs from the others in this book in that the weed isn't decarboxylized first, leading to a less-efficient THC infusion. It still produces a potent brew, though, so don't overdo it. This is the perfect drink to share with friends.

2 cups **water**

1 ounce **weed**

4 cups **full-fat, or whole, milk**

2 tablespoons **chopped almonds**

2 teaspoons **grenadine** (pomegranate syrup)

½ cup **sugar**

1 teaspoon **ground ginger**

½ teaspoon **garam masala** (Indian spice blend made with coriander, cumin, turmeric, etc.)

2 tablespoons **coconut milk**

1. Simmer the weed in the water in a small pan for 10 minutes.

2. Strain the water into another pan with a sieve, retaining the boiled weed leaves.

3. With a mortar and pestle (or in a bowl), grind these leaves up with about 2 tablespoons of the milk to make a paste. Drain off the milk into the pan of water.

4. Add the chopped almonds to the paste and mix together, then add another 2 tablespoons of milk, mix it all together, then drain off the milk into the pan again (use the sieve to stop little bits of leaf from falling in). Repeat this step several times, until you have used all the milk in pounding the leaf.

5. Add the grenadine, sugar, ginger, garam masala, and coconut milk to the pan of milk and water. Heat gently, until the milk simmers, then remove and let it cool down.

6. When cool, chill the lassi for a couple of hours, then serve in small glasses.

Bhang lassi

If you've ever had a cooling lassi to accompany a spicy Indian meal, you know how delicious this traditional dairy drink can be; and bhang lassi is something a little bit special in the world of cannabis cuisine. It's been consumed in India for hundreds—possibly thousands—of years, and is an element of many religious and cultural practices as well as being a refreshing, buzzy high. It's often drunk during *Holi*, the festival of colors, and *Maha Shivaratri*, a festival held in honor of the Hindu god Shiva. Across India, but especially in the north, it's widely available.

Smoothies

You can give any kind of smoothie a nice mellow by adding some Cannabis sugar (see page 181) into the mixer when you blend it. Initially try about 1 teaspoon for each portion. Classic ingredients include almond milk, fruit juice, banana, peach, mango, avocado, berries, spinach, chia seeds, yogurt, pineapple… the only limit is your imagination.

Green smoothie

Combine 9 fluid ounces of your preferred milk, ¼ teaspoon spirulina, a pinch of cinnamon, 1 banana, 1 handful of spinach, 1¾ ounces broccoli, and 1 teaspoon Cannabis sugar into a blender and blend until smooth.

Fruit smoothie

Combine 9 fluid ounces of water, segments from 1 orange, 1 large carrot, a few frozen mango and peach chunks, and 1 teaspoon Cannabis sugar into a blender and blend until smooth.

Snacks & Bakes

Bringing new meaning to the expression "high tea," these snacks will give you a lift at any time of day and keep you happy for longer...

Cannachoc-dipped strawberries

This is possibly the most indulgent way there is to deliver a hit.

4 ounces **dark chocolate** (70 percent cocoa solids)— your basic bar of Hershey's won't do the strawberries justice

4 teaspoons **Cannabutter** (see page 176), for a low dose

1 pound ripe **strawberries**

1. Place a glass bowl over a pan of boiling water, making the sure the base doesn't touch the water, break the chocolate into it, and stir with a wooden spoon until the chocolate has melted. Then mix through the cannabutter, ensuring that it is evenly distributed in the chocolate.

2. Holding them by their leafy tops, dip the strawberries into the chocolate, then place them on a sheet of baking parchment to set. Refrigerating them will give the chocolate a crunch!

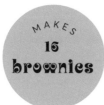

Hash brownies

If you've read this far in a book such as this, it's likely that you already know your way around a hash brownie! A classic, tasty way to deliver a hit of weedy goodness, they can easily be shared, make a great icebreaker at parties, and are cheap to make. If you've got leftovers, they freeze perfectly, too.

8 ounces **dark chocolate** (70 percent cocoa solids)

7 ounces **butter**

1 cup **sugar**

½ cup **Cannabis sugar** (see page 181)

1 cup **all-purpose flour**

3 large beaten **free-range eggs**

1. Preheat the oven to 340°F.

2. Place a glass bowl over a pan of boiling water, making the sure the base doesn't touch the water, break the chocolate into it and melt with the butter. Stir in the sugar, Cannabis sugar, the flour, and the eggs. Mix the batter until smooth, then spoon it into a greased 9-inch square baking pan.

3. Bake for 30 minutes: the top should be flaky and dry, the inside moist. Let the brownies rest overnight before slicing into sixteen chunks, each of which will have one modest dose.

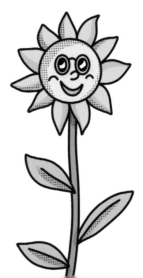

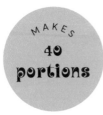

Cannabis caramels

Another classic candy, but a little trickier to make; only attempt these if you have a cooking thermometer.

2 cups **sugar**

1 cup **brown sugar**

1 cup **corn syrup**

1 cup **evaporated milk**

1 pint **heavy cream**

8 ounces **butter**

2 ounces **Cannabis sugar or Cannabutter** (see pages 181 or 176), for twenty low doses

2 teaspoons **vanilla extract**

1. Grease a 12 x 15-inch baking pan.

2. In a medium saucepan, combine the sugars, corn syrup, evaporated milk, heavy cream, and butter. Dose with the Cannabis sugar or Cannabutter, as you prefer. Warm the pan over medium heat, stirring all the time and monitoring the temperature with the thermometer. At 250°F, turn off the heat. Stir in the vanilla extract, then carefully pour the mixture into the prepared baking pan and let it cool and solidify.

3. When cooled, cut the caramel into forty portions, noting that two will provide a low dose. Store covered in the fridge for up to two weeks.

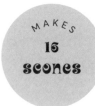
Cannabis scones

These are an easy bake, but one that you really want to eat fresh—they lose that delicious moistness after a day or two.

2 cups **all-purpose flour**

4 teaspoons **baking powder**

1 teaspoon **salt**

½ cup **butter or shortening**

3–4 teaspoons **Cannabutter** (see page 176), for a low dose

¾ cup **milk**

1. Preheat the oven to 400°F.

2. Mix the flour with the baking powder and salt, then add the butter or shortening and the Cannabutter, and mix until it is the texture of crumbs. Then add the milk and knead to a soft dough. Roll out to about ½-inch thick, cut into circles, and bake for 12–15 minutes.

3. Serve with butter and honey, or, if you can get hold of some Devonshire (or clotted) cream, then make like a British aristocrat and apply a layer of that and a layer of strawberry jam.

Happy chocolate bars

For a discreet, portable happy meal, why not make your own cannabis chocolate bars? You're adding fat to the chocolate, so you need to use a brand that doesn't have much to start with. Place a glass bowl over a pan of boiling water, making sure the base doesn't touch the water, break 4 ounces dark chocolate (70 percent cocoa solids) into it, and stir until melted. Then stir through 4 teaspoons Cannabutter (see page 176), ensuring it is evenly mixed through the chocolate. Pour the chocolate into a mold or ice-cube tray or drip it onto baking parchment to make buttons. Place in the fridge to solidify.

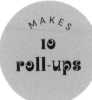
Happy fruit roll-ups

This one is really simple.

3 cups **strawberries or raspberries or blueberries** (or any mixture thereof)

2 tablespoons **Cannabis sugar** (see page 181)

2 tablespoons **lemon juice**

1. Preheat your oven to its lowest setting.

2. Blend the fruit with the Cannabis sugar and lemon juice. Blend them until the mixture is completely smooth.

3. Cover a baking sheet with plastic wrap, then spread the mixture out on top of it, as thin as it will go without forming holes (¼-inch thick or less). Put it into your oven and let it dehydrate for at least 4 hours—maybe more—until the middle isn't tacky any more, then you're done.

4. Use scissors to cut it into strips, then roll up. This recipe contains about ten low doses, so keep track of how many roll-ups you make from the batch.

Happy Pancakes

It's easy to make many pancakes in one batch, so this is a good option if you want to feed a few people. Add Cannabis oil (see page 175) to the batter—about 1 teaspoon per portion—and if you want a double hit, sprinkle with Cannabis sugar (see page 181) or spread a little Cannabutter (see page 176) over them when they're hot.

Oatmeal energy balls

Another option for on-the-go power-ups, these balls are super easy to make and you only have to wash up one bowl! These balls will have about four modest doses between them.

1¼ cups **rolled oats**

½ cup **peanut butter**

¼ cup **honey**

A pinch of **salt**

1 teaspoon **vanilla extract**

2–3 teaspoons
Cannabis sugar
(see page 181)

½ cup **dried fruit, dried berries, chocolate chips, chopped nuts, or seeds**

1. Mix the rolled oats with the peanut butter, honey, a pinch of salt, the vanilla extract, and cannabis sugar. Make sure the sugar is evenly mixed through. Then add your chosen dried fruit, dried berries, chocolate chips, chopped nuts, or seeds.

2. Place the mixture in the fridge for about an hour so that it sets and is easier to shape, then portion up and mix into balls of about 1 inch in diameter. If the mix is a little too sticky, roll it in some more oats to coat the balls.

3. Keep covered in the fridge for up to two weeks.

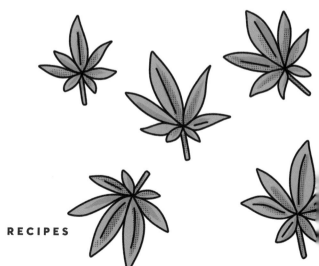

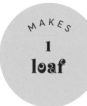

Marijuana banana bread

This feels almost as good to say as it does to eat! This will contain about 4–5 modest doses.

3 over-ripe **bananas**

1½ cups **all-purpose flour**

1 cup **sugar**

¼ cup **soft butter**

1 teaspoon **vanilla extract**

½ teaspoon **baking powder**

1 teaspoon **baking soda**

1 **free-range egg**

1 tablespoon **Cannabutter or Cannabis coconut oil** (see pages 176 or 182), plus extra for greasing

1. Preheat the oven to 350°F. Grease and line a 2-pound loaf pan.

2. Mash the bananas in a bowl and add the flour, sugar, soft butter, vanilla extract, baking powder, baking soda, and egg. Add the Cannabutter or Cannabis coconut oil. Mix well.

3. Pour into the loaf pan and bake for about 1 hour (or until a skewer inserted into the cake comes out clean).

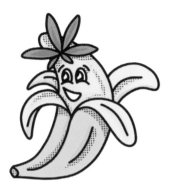

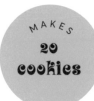

MAKES
20 cookies

Peanut butter cannacookies

Very, very simple to make, especially if you have a blender. This recipe yields around twenty cookies, each of which will have one modest dose.

½ cup **soft butter**

¼ cup **brown sugar**

½ cup **sugar**

¼ cup **Cannabis sugar**
(see page 181)

½ cup **peanut butter**

1 **free-range egg**

1 teaspoon **vanilla extract**

1½ cups **all-purpose flour**

½ teaspoon **baking powder**

½ teaspoon **salt**

1. Cream the butter with all the sugars. Mix or blend until the mixture is light and fluffy. Add the peanut butter, egg, and vanilla extract and mix together. Add the flour, baking powder, and salt. Mix into a smooth dough and roll out into a log. Chill this in the fridge for an hour.

2. Preheat the oven to 350°F.

3. Cut the log into twenty equal slices and lay out on a baking sheet lined with baking parchment. Use a fork to mark a pattern on the tops. Bake for about 10 minutes, until the cookies are golden. Remove and leave to cool for at least 5 minutes.

Cannabis and chocolate ice cream

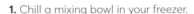

This will yield about ten servings of low to moderate strength.

One 14-ounce **can sweetened condensed milk**

½ cup **cocoa powder**

3 tablespoons **Cannabis sugar** (see page 181)

1 teaspoon **vanilla extract**

2 cups **heavy cream**

1. Chill a mixing bowl in your freezer.

2. Pour the condensed milk into a bowl with the cocoa powder, Cannabis sugar, and vanilla extract. Whisk until evenly mixed.

3. Take the bowl out of your freezer, then use it to whisk the heavy cream: the cream is ready when stiff peaks form easily. Add half the whipped cream to the sweetened condensed milk mixture, gently folding it in with a rubber spatula. Then pour that mixture back into the bowl of whipped cream, folding it gently until well blended. Be careful not to overmix it—you don't want the whipped cream to collapse. Pour into a Tupperware container and put into the freezer immediately. It should be solid in 2–3 hours.

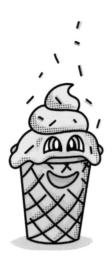

Happy oat bars

Known in the U.K. as "flapjacks," these oat bars are super-easy and cheap to make and are sustaining, healthy snacks.

5 ounces **butter**

²/₃ cup **brown sugar**

2 tablespoons **corn syrup or molasses**

A pinch of **salt**

3 tablespoons **Cannabutter** (see page 176)

10 ounces **oatmeal**

1. Preheat the oven to 380°F. Lightly butter an 8 x 8-inch baking pan.

2. Melt the butter in a small pan over low heat, then mix in the brown sugar, corn syrup or molasses, a pinch of salt, and the Cannabutter. Tip the hot mixture into a bowl with the oatmeal and stir together with a wooden spoon until the texture and color are even.

3. Scoop the mixture into the prepared pan. Press into the corners with the back of a spoon so the mixture is flat and, using a knife tip, score into sixteen squares. Bake for around 15 minutes until golden brown.

Happy waffles

Whether you are serving these as an indulgent brunch or a delightful dessert, just stir some Cannabis oil (see page 175) into the batter before you pour it onto the waffle iron—about 1 teaspoon per portion. Top with whipped cream, ice cream, chopped fruit, and chocolate sauce...

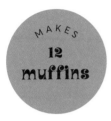

Marijuana muffins

This makes about twelve plain muffins: feel free to add choc chips, blueberries, cinnamon, fruit, or whatever else you like to the basic mix!

2 cups **all-purpose flour**

1 teaspoon **baking powder**

1 teaspoon **baking soda**

½ teaspoon **salt**

4 ounces softened **unsalted butter**

2½ tablespoons **Cannabutter** (see page 176)

¾ cup **white sugar**

2 large **eggs**

½ cup **plain yogurt**

2 teaspoons **vanilla extract**

¼ cup **milk**

1. Preheat the oven to 400°F, and lightly oil a twelve-cup muffin pan or add paper cupcake liners.

2. In a large bowl, stir together the flour, baking powder, baking soda, and salt. In a second bowl, cream together the butter, Cannabutter, sugar, eggs, yogurt, and vanilla extract. Mix this into the dry ingredients, then stir through the milk.

3. Pour the batter into the prepared muffin pan and bake for 5 minutes. Then reduce the oven temperature to 350°F, and bake for another 15–20 minutes or until a skewer poked into the muffins comes out clean.

Choc chip cannacookies

Another sweet treat that every self-respecting cannabis chef needs to master. Aim to make about twenty cookies: each one will then have one modest dose.

6 ounces **butter**

2 ounces **Cannabutter** (see page 176)

7 ounces **white sugar**

7 ounces **brown sugar**

2 **large eggs**

2 teaspoons **vanilla extract**

1 teaspoon **baking soda**

½ teaspoon **salt**

3 cups **all-purpose flour**

8 ounces **milk or dark chocolate chips**

1. Preheat the oven to 350°F.

2. Cream together the butter, Cannabutter, and both sugars until smooth. Beat in the eggs one at a time, then add the vanilla extract.

3. In another bowl, mix together the baking soda, salt, flour, and chocolate chips. Add all the dry ingredients to the wet and stir together until you have an even batter.

4. With a ladle, spoon onto an ungreased baking sheet, one dollop per cookie, and bake for about 10 minutes in the oven, or until the cookies' edges are nicely browned.

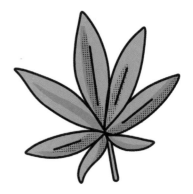

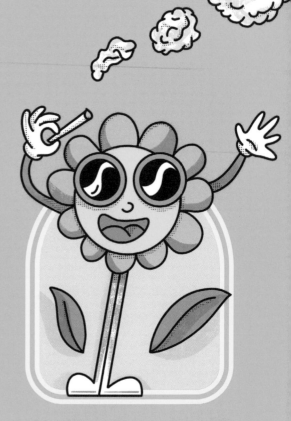

Horticultural Smokes

There are good reasons why people get into gardening as they get older: it's relaxing, natural, stimulating, and a great hobby to share with friends and loved ones. Remind you of anything? Growing your own weed is becoming ever more popular, and today there are a host of online resources and stores that will supply you with seeds and everything you need to grow them. Whatever the strain, whatever the balance of THC to CBD, however you smoke it, the most satisfying grass is the grass you've grown yourself. It's also cheap, productive, and gardening itself is a highly therapeutic activity. Here's a quick-start guide to how to go about it. Be warned, your home will smell dank with the plants—so don't grow your own if that's going to be a problem…

There are good reasons why people get into gardening as they get older: it's relaxing, natural, and stimulating.

Whatever the strain, whatever the balance of THC to CBD, however you smoke it, the most satisfying grass is the grass you've grown yourself.

Pick your seed

Get hold of some feminized seed—this guarantees that all your plants will be female. (Yes, you read that right, you get male and female cannabis plants, but only the female kind produce smokable buds.) If you live in a hot climate, choose a hybrid with more *sativa* to it; if cooler, then an *indica*. Your first plant should be forgiving and easy for beginners to grow.

Planting

If you live in a warm climate, then you need to find a nice sunny and private spot where you can tend and water your bud. You want your plant to get as much noon sun as possible and stay within 55 and 86°F. A light breeze is good for ventilation and plant health. Plant your seed after the last frost, in the ground or a 5–10-gallon container, with a nice crumbly loam soil and some fertilizer (horse muck is great, if you can get it).

Nurture

Keep moist, but not overwatered, and watch the plant grow! Toward the end of the growing season, she will start to send out buds—this is what you are looking for.

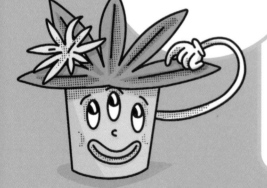

Home hydroponics

Growing indoors is more expensive and requires specialist equipment. Your home will smell, you will need to give over a room to the plants, and you don't have that glorious organic naturalness. But… you will get a reliable, high-quality harvest.

Curing

This crucial two-stage process removes the moisture from the buds and makes them truly dank. You want to cure slowly, to maximize levels of THC, give your weed a long shelf life, and also to decompose the chlorophyll and plant sugars—which is what makes a bad joint taste so harsh on the throat.

First, you dry out the whole plant—so you need a dark room, humidity around 50 percent, and a fan circulating the air. When the plant is dry (after about a week, its flowers will feel a little crunchy, and twigs will easily snap), pick the buds and transfer them to airtight jars. Pack loosely—don't crush the buds. For one week, open the jar to air it about four times a day, for a few minutes each time. After a week, open once every other day. Continue like this for at least three weeks—but feel free to go longer—it may well give you a more mellow smoke.

Home harvest festival

Celebrate your harvest with its own fall festival. Invite some friends over, get a bong ready, maybe decarboxylate some of your buds and bake with them…

Storing for long life

Don't freeze! It will reduce the THC content of your bud. Instead, keep it in a jar, in a dark place, between 60 and 70°F. Don't let it dry out completely and don't let it get damp or moldy.

Hidden glade

If you are lucky enough to live near the woods, why not find a clearing and sow a whole bunch of seeds— mixed male and female. If they take and reproduce, you'll have a magical hidden glade of free weed that you can harvest and share.

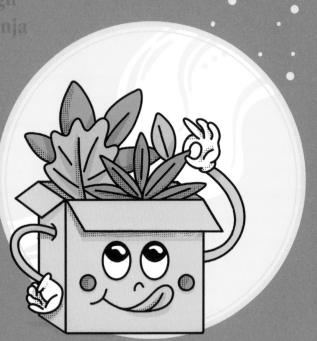

Strains

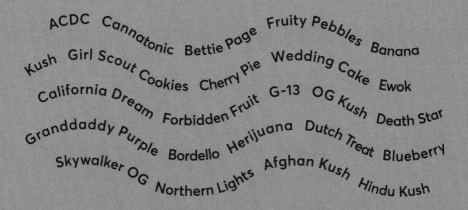

ACDC Cannatonic Bettie Page Fruity Pebbles Banana Kush Girl Scout Cookies Cherry Pie Wedding Cake Ewok California Dream Forbidden Fruit G-13 OG Kush Death Star Granddaddy Purple Bordello Herijuana Dutch Treat Blueberry Skywalker OG Northern Lights Afghan Kush Hindu Kush

In the old days, most of us used to smoke what we could get. If it was perfectly cured bud in excellent condition, fantastic; if it was old dry shwag and stem, well, it would

They all look beautiful, smell aromatic, and have been carefully raised.

have to do. Today, the wide variety of strains on sale in a licensed dispensary can be bewildering—they all look beautiful, smell aromatic, and have been carefully raised, so how can you choose which bud will be the best use of your buck? In this section, we put your choice into context, looking at the differences between *sativa, indica,* and hybrid strains, before picking out fifty that are definitely worth exploring.

Sativa, Indica & the Spectrum of Hybrids

There are three subspecies of cannabis plants that have useful quantities of THC, CBD, and related cannabinoids and terpenes. Of these, one (*ruderalis*) is small and comparatively weak. It grows in the wild in northern India, where it is a source of hand-rolled hashish, but you're unlikely to come across it in your dispensary. That leaves *sativa*, which grows in the wild in North Africa, Turkey, and Asia, and *indica*, most common in Afghanistan, India, and Pakistan. (Note, though, that cannabis is a pretty tough plant and has been spread by human traffic throughout the world, so wild cannabis plants of either strain are not an unusual sight across Europe, Asia, and the Americas. Such strains are called "landraces" and many of them are excellent smokes.) What does this mean for the smoker? There are significant differences between *sativa* and *indica*: by and large, *sativa* strains are high in THC (the fun compound), while *indica* has less THC and a higher amount of CBD—which is responsible for most of marijuana's medicinal benefits.

To complicate matters, *sativa* and *indica* breed happily with each other, and the resulting hybrid strains contain varying amounts of the different terpenes and other cannabinoids, meaning that you can find a strain at any point of the spectrum from pure *sativa* to pure *indica*.

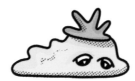

What **sativa** brings to a strain	What **indica** brings to a strain
Euphoria	Tranquility and relaxation
A "head high"	A "body high"
Alertness	Intensified appetite
Creativity	Sleepiness
Energy boost	Pain relief

You may find that *sativa* works best in the daytime and *indica* late at night. To follow is a journey along the spectrum, with fifty strains listed from pure *sativa* to pure *indica*. The order is not necessarily exact: we are talking cannabis growers, here, after all. Note that this does not cover their medicinal properties; if you want an authoritative guide to medical marijuana, you should consult a specialist guide like Michael Backes' *Cannabis Pharmacy*.

The THC content below is an approximate maximum: professionally grown weed should be around the level cited, but much depends on climate, care, storage, and curing, so your bud may well be less potent. Where significant, CBD content is included: this is harder for growers to control, though, so check with your dispensary if this is what you're looking for in particular. Assume that if it's not mentioned, CBD levels are negligible.

(100% S) Hawaiian Snow—A multiaward winner, heavy on the THC—up to 24 percent—and notorious for provoking giggling fits, with an energetic high that subsides into dreamy happiness.

(100% S) Durban Poison—A strain that emerged in the wild in South Africa, this is almost pure THC at high levels—around 18 percent—and minimal CBD. A sweet, fruity smoke, with very energetic properties, it's known as the espresso of bud.

(95% S) Lamb's Bread—This Jamaican landrace strain (taken to the island by Indian indentured laborers in the nineteenth century) played an important role in the history of cannabis and music alike, as it was a favorite smoke of Bob Marley and a host of other reggae musicians. With THC of around 18 percent and a powerful, uplifting high, it's not hard to understand why…

(80% S) Haze—Rumored to have originated in Santa Cruz, this was the dominant strain of the Californian 1960s. Widely hybridized, it's deservedly still popular in its original form and is a great smoke to share: you'll be chatty, energetic, yet enjoy full-body relaxation. THC levels vary from 18 percent up to a whopping 27 percent, so don't overdo it—paranoia is also a recognized side-effect.

(80% S) Haze Berry—The "Berry" refers to the sweetness, and this hybrid promises a long-lasting, creative high—some say it's great if you want to "get things done." Approximately 20 percent THC, with low CBD.

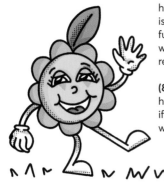

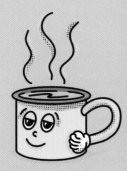

Amnesia Mac Ganja

(80% S) Amnesia Haze—A complicated hybrid with origins in *sativas* from Hawaii, Thailand, Cambodia, California, and Jamaica, this is one of the strongest buds you'll come across, with 24 percent THC typical and just a little CBD to bring the mellow. Euphoria, energy, and focus are common effects.

(80% S) Strawberry Cough—Originally hybridized by Kyle Kushman, a former cultivation editor at *High Times*, this can be a harsh smoke (hence the name) but is famous for the focus it brings to intellectual activity and brain work—and its long-lasting high. Typically 18 percent THC in content.

(80% S) Amnesia Mac Ganja—A multiaward winner, this strain has long been popular in Amsterdam's coffee shops thanks to its herby, spicy flavor and more than respectable THC content of 22 percent. A serene, happy high.

(80% S) Chernobyl—A distinctive aroma of lime sherbet precedes a smoke that isn't overpowering (THC clocks in at a moderate 17 percent or so) and a floaty, happy high that is less about euphoria than relaxation.

(80% S) Sour Diesel—With its origins lost in the smoky mists of time, no one knows what strains gave rise to this potent—very strong—hybrid. With a raw, distinctive taste (some find it too harsh and complain of a cotton mouth afterward), this is a stimulating high delivering 22 percent of THC right where it matters.

(80% S) Maui Waui—From Hawaii, as you'd expect, this strain has been popular since the 1960s and, like many "heritage" strains, isn't overpoweringly strong. Moderate 17 percent THC will get you cheery, buzzing, and clear-headed. A fun smoke to enjoy in company.

(75% S) Laughing Buddha—This hybrid of the best of Thai and Jamaican *sativa* strains will, as promised, bring on the giggles. A touch of CBD (1 percent) and moderate THC (18 percent) mean that this won't have you doing anything stupid, but you'll be talkative, happy, sociable, and great company.

(75% S) Moby Dick—You'd expect that a strain named for a combative whale would be strong and that's the case here: up to 27 percent THC in the bud and a powerful high the result. Can be trippy, with citrus notes to the smoke.

(75% S) Shining Silver Haze—Descended from Skunk, one of the most notorious *indica* strains of the 1990s, this offers a very different high: physical, happy, and clear-headed. Up to 21 percent THC with low CBD and a popular aroma.

(75% S) Gorilla Glue #4—A complicated hybrid that is one of the strongest buds on the market—THC levels can reach a staggering 32 percent. That means it might not be for everyone (you shouldn't really attempt to do much else, if you get seriously into the GG4) but it has won multiple awards, and the plant has been described as "some trichomes with a bunch of buds, leaves and stalks sticking to them."

(75% S) Harlequin—A strain that's a favorite with medicinal marijuana users: approximately 9 percent CBD and 5 percent THC deliver balanced relaxation and pain relief with a nicely enhanced mood on the side. Focus and energy are also reported effects, making this a great strain to help you get on with your day.

(70% S) Red Dragon—This sweet-smoked hybrid is a real joy, known for a high that opens with an energetic uplift and then settles for a few hours of pleasing stonedness. Not overly powerful, with THC around 16 percent, Red Dragon may well bring on the munchies.

(70% S) Acapulco Gold—A Mexican landrace, this has been deservedly popular for decades: a cheerful, upbeat smoke with sweet burnt-sugar and nutmeg notes and around 19 percent THC.

(65% S) Hulkberry—Hugely popular on both sides of the Atlantic, Hulkberry is a monster with up to 27 percent THC. Go easy with it, therefore, but enjoy the ride as you do: fruity, with a powerful mental lift that lasts a long time, this will boost you nicely.

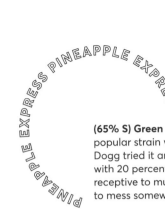

PINEAPPLE EXPRESS PINEAPPLE EXPRESS PINEAPPLE EXPRESS

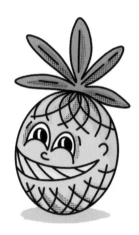

(65% S) Green Crack—Originating in Athens, Georgia, this popular strain was originally called "Cush" or "Kush" until Snoop Dogg tried it and renamed it on the spot. A great daytime high with 20 percent THC, this is an energetic high that leaves you receptive to music, movies, or the arts in general and is reported to mess somewhat with your sense of time passing.

(65% S) AK-47—A multiaward-winning giant of international competition, this is an herbal, happy smoke, with THC around 17 percent and a 1.5 percent CBD that takes a little of the edge off, yielding a relaxing, mellow high for the head.

(60% S) Green Crack Punch—With a high that moves from uplifting to creative to relaxed to lazy, this is a best-of-both worlds strain that can be about 20 percent THC.

(60% S) Pineapple Express—A long-time favorite in the cafés of Amsterdam, this is a great daytime smoke that sparks conversation and creativity alike—a great social smoke—and at 24 percent THC, pretty strong. Users report high productivity!

(60% S) El Patron—This brings the buzz to body and mind and has won the Highlife Cup as a result. A distinctive mixture of flavorsome terpenes, along with 22 percent THC, makes it particularly popular among chefs.

(60% S) White Widow—One of the most striking-looking of all cannabis plants, this produces buds that are so heavy in white trichomes that they almost resemble snowballs. They, in turn, reliably yield THC at 20 percent or more, and that, in turn, makes this one a perennial favorite in Dutch coffee shops. It hits fast, with a chatty, euphoric head high.

(55% S) Jack Herer—With high levels of THC (around 20 percent) and low levels of CBD (1–2 percent), this is named for the author of *The Emperor Wears No Clothes* and is certainly a fitting tribute. Users note a blissful happiness and cooling sensation.

(50% S/50% I) Blue Dream—A perfect half-and-half hybrid, Blue Dream is distinguished by its high levels of CBD, with 2 percent making this a versatile medical marijuana strain. On top of that, you have 20 percent THC, giving you a great head rush: focus, determination, and new ideas will follow. This mellows into a calm, relaxed hour or two—no wonder it's popular.

(50% S/50% I) ACDC—One of the few strains on this list to have higher CBD content (18 percent) than THC (2 percent), this is a smoke that is intensely relaxing, with great medicinal properties, but hardly any psychoactive ones. So, no giggles, but a deep chill.

(50% S/50% I) Cannatonic—Another 50/50 hybrid with high CBD, this was one of the first strains to reliably bear more CBD (up to 12 percent) than THC (6 percent), so it's less about the high than the relaxation. Known for the sense of clarity, this is a smoke that will relax you profoundly—without locking you to the couch.

(50% S/50% I) Bettie Page—Similar in profile to the other half-and-half hybrids already mentioned, this is not a strong bud (THC at 14 percent, CBD at 2 percent), but it delivers a gentle mellow that is both therapeutic and enjoyable.

(55% I) Fruity Pebbles—A mid-strength strain (18 percent) that is often recommended for occasional or beginner smokers: users refer to a mental buzz that can help you focus and create. Fun, without being out of control.

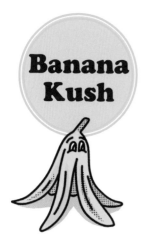

(60% I) Banana Kush—A very nicely balanced bud, and phenomenally strong, at 27 percent THC. Yes, it does smell and taste of bananas, with a smooth, creative, uplifting, full-body high that makes it a popular smoke for artists.

(60% I) Girl Scout Cookies—A cross between two other beloved strains on this chart, OG Kush and Durban Poison, this Cannabis Cup winner is a lovely late-night smoke. THC levels at 25 percent or more and 1 percent CBD deliver a best-of-both-worlds smoke with euphoria, deep relaxation, and the munchies.

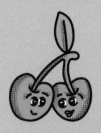

(60% I) Cherry Pie—Recommended as an aphrodisiac, this tasty strain is popular in dispensaries and is good at all times, but especially the evening. With 20 percent THC, it brings a slow high that peaks after a few minutes, with relaxation slipping into calm analysis and connection-forming. The epitome of a well-balanced hybrid: if you could only have one strain on hand, Cherry Pie would be an excellent choice.

(60% I) Wedding Cake—A 25 percent THC hybrid that includes some Girl Scout Cookies in the mix, this strain takes you on a mellow journey, with a fast, sparky high followed by a long, smooth ride down. Some find the smoke harsh, but many praise it for delivering a paranoia-free, relaxed, calming high.

(60% I) Ewok—Known for being a spacey, cerebral smoke, Ewok is a prize-winning hybrid from the Seattle area with 19 percent THC. It is profoundly relaxing, with a heavy, herbal smoke and a full-body hit. Also known as Alien Walker.

(70% I) California Dream—The plants of this Mexican–Afghan hybrid can grow to a towering 8 feet tall, but it's no brute to smoke: it's popular for its social vibe, and smokers note focused happiness. At 24 percent THC, that's no surprise…

(70% I) Forbidden Fruit—Notable for a smooth burn and calming, head-downward relaxation that makes it an excellent late-night smoke and great to reduce anxiety and bring on a long, sound night's sleep. At 26 percent THC, you don't need more than a few tokes to set yourself on your way.

(70% I) G-13—The "G" stands for government, apparently. The urban legend is that this hard-hitter was hybridized at the University of Mississippi with the help of the CIA and FBI. Mmmm, right. Don't let that shaky backstory put you off: this is a fan favorite, with a full-body lazy hit that relaxes you profoundly and delivers a sleepy euphoria. That'll be the work of the 18 percent THC, not the Pentagon…

(75% I) OG Kush—Try this one if you're restless and want a nice woody aroma in your smoke. With 19 percent THC, it's mellow, and will set you on the path to dreamland and a good night's sleep.

(75% I) Death Star—Like its *Star Wars* namesake, this is slow-moving, heavy, and fearsomely powerful. Don't be deceived if the first few puffs don't get you anywhere: that high will be along in a minute, and then you'll be stuck in a slow orbit around a forest moon… Heavy on the THC (20 percent or more) and with CBD to calm you at the same time, this will set you up perfectly for a couch-based movie marathon.

(75% I) Granddaddy Purple—A heavy, heavy *indica* that is great for late nights, although more powerful than its 20 percent THC content might suggest; you may wake up on the couch in the small hours, having dropped off after your evening smoke…

(75% I) Bordello—Don't smoke this if you need to get stuff done. Unless you count "experiencing a paralyzing sense of euphoria" as getting stuff done, which is a valid lifestyle choice, after all… This strain is known to vary in strength considerably, but can hit 22 percent THC, so go easy on it to begin. It will hit you in the head first, then spread to the body and give you an all-over glow.

(80% I) Herijuana—Carefully hybridized, this is the love child of Petrolia Headstash and Killer New Haven and delivers a whopping 25 percent THC in a typically *indican* knockout bud. You will be sedated; a majority of users found this a sleepy smoke, but intensely relaxing, too. Many also report a tingling sensation, or meditative thoughts.

(80% I) Dutch Treat—Mmmmm, this *is* the smell of Amsterdam. Intense eucalyptus aromas foreshadow a rapid head high that is pure euphoria. Happiness, relaxation, all the good stuff is delivered by 19 percent THC, and with a delicious smoke as well.

(80% I) Blueberry—A classic *indica*-dominant strain that has lent its fragrant qualities to many hybrids over the years and won the Best Strain award at the 2000 *High Times* Cannabis Cup. At 16 percent THC, it's not strong, but the high is popular and very, very relaxing.

(85% I) Skywalker OG—This hits you fast and will leave you happy, hungry, and glued to the couch. With a THC content of around 20 percent, it's not a knockout, more of a steady sedative, and is a great wind-down at the end of a hard day.

(95% I) Northern Lights—One of the purest *indica* strains out there, this is also one of the most popular. Rumored to originate from Seattle, it balances 18 percent THC with about 1 percent CBD and promises a relaxed euphoria, earthy aroma, and sleepiness.

(95% I) Afghan Kush—The nearest thing to smoking hash, this 15 percent THC strain grows in the wild in Afghanistan and has a piney, resinous aroma. Not the smoothest or strongest smoke, but it is excellent for your aches and pains, and a nice relaxed high will creep up on you over a few minutes.

(100% I) Hindu Kush—A real knockout drop, this gives you a lovely soporific euphoria that may leave you feeling somewhat sedated… Modest 18 percent THC with 1 percent CBD, and reputed to originate in the mountains of the same name that run from Afghanistan into Pakistan.

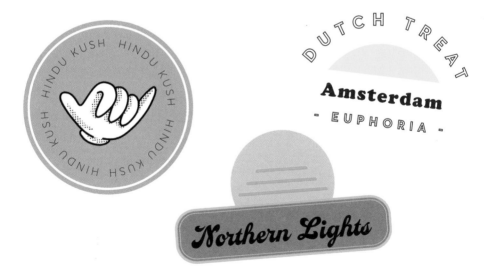

Index

Acknowledgments

My sincerest thanks go to Helen Rochester, for entertaining the idea of this title; my neighbors, especially Neon, for regularly wafting inspirational smoke through the open window while I wrote; Caitlin Doyle, for burning the midnight oil to turn the manuscript into the volume that you hold now; and more than anyone, Jules, for being Jules.

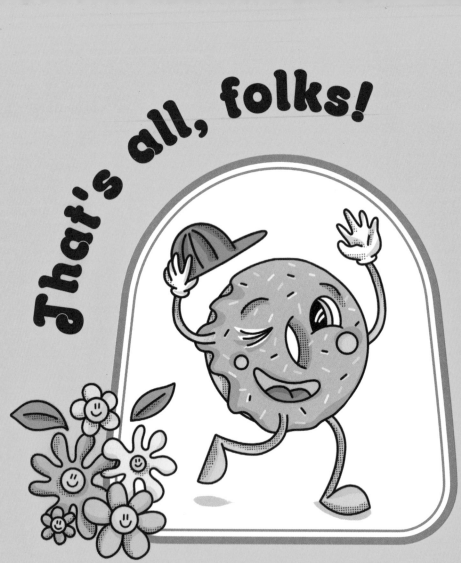